CRISIS CENTER/HOTLINE

CRISIS CENTER/HOTLINE
A Guidebook to Beginning and Operating

Edited by

URSULA DELWORTH, Ph.D.
EDWARD H. RUDOW, Ph.D.
JANET TAUB

Colorado State University
Fort Collins, Colorado

With a Foreword by

Weston Morrill, Ph.D.

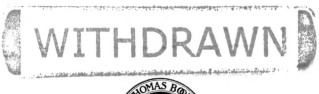
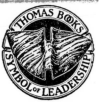

CHARLES C THOMAS • PUBLISHER
Springfield • *Illinois* • *U.S.A.*

Published and Distributed Throughout the World by

CHARLES C THOMAS • PUBLISHER

BANNERSTONE HOUSE

301-327 East Lawrence Avenue, Springfield, Illinois, U.S.A.

© *1972, by* CHARLES C THOMAS • PUBLISHER

ISBN 0-398-02561-4

Library of Congress Catalog Card Number: 72-79187

With THOMAS BOOKS *careful attention is given to all details of manufacturing and design. It is the Publisher's desire to present books that are satisfactory as to their physical qualities and artistic possibilities and appropriate for their particular use.* THOMAS BOOKS *will be true to those laws of quality that assure a good name and good will.*

Printed in the United States of America
PP-22

To
LLOYD KELLEY

*the first director of RoadHouse, whose laughter eased
some of the growing pains, whose own caring created
caring in all of us.*

CONTRIBUTORS

URSULA DELWORTH, PH.D.: *Assistant Professor of Psychology, Colorado State University; Senior Psychologist, Colorado State University Counseling Center.*

NORMAN L. FARBEROW, PH.D.: *Clinical Associate Professor of Psychiatry and Psychology, University of Southern California School of Medicine; Co-director of Suicide Prevention Center, Los Angeles, California.*

BERNIE GEBHARDT: *Paraprofessional, Fort Collins Drug Education Project; Formerly Director of "The Point," Fort Collins Drug Crisis Center.*

CHARLOTTE GREENFIELD, J.D.: *Assistant Human Relations Executive, Colorado State University; Member, New York State Bar Association.*

SAM M. HEILIG, M.S.W.: *Executive Director and Director of Training, Suicide Prevention Center, Los Angeles, California.*

JOHN E. HINKLE, PH.D.: *Associate Professor of Psychology, Colorado State University; Associate Director, Colorado State University Counseling Center.*

ROBERT E. LITMAN, M.D.: *Chief Psychiatrist and Co-project Director, Suicide Prevention Center, Los Angeles, California.*

MARV MOORE, PH.D.: *Assistant Director, Colorado State University Counseling Center; Chairman of Board of Directors, Fort Collins Drug Education Project.*

EDWARD H. RUDOW, PH.D.: *Director, Fort Collins Drug Education Project.*

DAVID W. SMART, PH.D.: *Assistant Professor, College Student Personnel Work Department; University of Northern Colorado; Psychologist, UNC Counseling Center*

PENFIELD W. TATE, J.D.: *Human Relations Executive, Colorado State University.*

JANET TAUB: *Paraprofessional Advisor-Director, Campus Crisis Center, Colorado State University.*

FOREWORD

T HE development of hundreds of crisis and hotline centers in cities and universities throughout the United States demonstrate some important directions and happenings in the mental health field. The crisis centers reflect an important change in the presentation and delivery of services to those in need as well as a significant change in the personnel who deliver those services.

Crisis centers reflect a change in the delivery of services in that their intent is to provide services that are easily accessible to large numbers of people. In addition, the intent is to have these services available whenever people are in crisis rather than only during the traditional 8:00 A.M. to 5:00 P.M. schedule. These centers thus represent an important shift in the delivery and availability of services to those in need.

Another important trend in the mental health field which the crisis centers demonstrate is the inclusion of nonprofessionals in the delivery of services. The majority of crisis centers are manned by lay volunteers who are given training specific to the tasks they perform. Too often professionals fail to fully appreciate and utilize the skills and competencies of lay volunteers. Perhaps as professionals we are overly concerned about the preservation of our professional mystique or overly dependent upon our graduate training.

This is an important book for those who are involved in the establishment and operation of such centers. The book provides practical information about the day-to-day operation of a crisis center based on the experience of establishing and running such a center. The book provides insights and experiences by both professionals and volunteer students and thus provides a model for the inclusion of paraprofessionals in the mental health field.

The value of this book is not limited to those involved in the establishment of crisis centers. There are source materials which would benefit many lay and professional mental health workers in other than the crisis calling center. The chapter on drugs, for example, would be valuable for any who are working in settings which bring them in contact with individuals with drug and drug-related problems.

In *Crisis Center Hotline A Guidebook to Beginning and Operating,* the authors have provided a practical, sensible, and usable guide for any who are involved in the process of establishing and operating such a center. Their effort in providing the results of their experiences for others to profit and build upon could have far-reaching effects in terms of the number of individuals who might have available to them effective services to meet their needs in time of crisis.

WESTON H. MORRILL
Associate Professor Psychology
Colorado State University

PREFACE

IN the past few years there has been a tremendous increase in the number of crisis center/hotline operations which have opened across the country. Some of these centers are limited in scope, while others are quite inclusive, offering a number of different services under one roof. Many are strictly referral agents; others handle crises or disseminate information themselves. Examples of some of the services offered are suicide prevention, drug information and crisis intervention, draft information, interpersonal relation problem-solving, medical clinics, crash pads, activity information, legal information, emergency transportation, employment information, and such. *The Exchange,* a crisis center/hotline newsletter, published by the Youth Emergency Service program in Minneapolis, reports that copies of their publication are sent to five hundred such centers and another two hundred are sent to other interested parties. This figure suggests a very conservative estimate of the number of centers which now exist.

Because we are associated with RoadHouse, the crisis calling center at Colorado State University, we are constantly receiving requests from other existing centers and also from people interested in opening centers. These people are usually looking for some type of guide to forming or operating a center. Many centers have outlines of their own operations, but often these are sketchy in detail and are limited to the needs of that particular center. Because of this, we decided that a general guide to operating a crisis center is needed both for those who are contemplating beginning a crisis center/hotline and those who are already operating one. In writing and editing this book we drew not only upon our own experiences, but those of other centers, using information and materials received from them over the past two years. In addition, we incorporated knowledge and suggestions from a number of conferences we have attended. We have tried to keep the book general, so that it can serve as a guide for the many different types of centers which are in need of some basic information. It should be realized, however, that each center has its own needs, and the suggestions offered are not meant as absolutes nor exhaustive, but rather as ideas to be modified and expanded as may be warranted.

The book itself has chapters dealing with such issues as how to physically operate a center, how to select and train workers, how to develop and maintain cohesion among the staff. There is a chapter offering advice on financing, another on legal considerations to be taken into account, and one on how to evaluate the center's operation. We have included one chapter dealing with a study on the psychological makeup of volunteers, to give an indication as to which people are most likely to become volunteers, and two chapters dealing with two major services which are offered by a large number of centers: suicide prevention and drug information and crisis intervention. These two chapters were included because of the concern a number of people have in handling these situations and also because they can serve as general guides in dealing with other problems.

The authors of the various chapters in the book were chosen because of their expertise and familiarity with the area of which they wrote. We feel that each chapter in and of itself contains worthwhile suggestions and can be read independently of the other chapters. However, if the most benefit is to be derived from the book, it should be read in its entirety.

Ursula Delworth
Edward H. Rudow
Janet Taub

ACKNOWLEDGMENTS

WE wish to express a note of appreciation to the many people who helped in the preparation of this book. The following persons spent many hours in reading rough drafts of the various chapters and offering helpful comments and suggestions: Gail Steiger, James and Sally Taub, Carol Geer, Grant Sherwood and Darlene Hinkle. Dr. Glenn C. Dildine certainly deserves mention for his assistance in the preparation of the chapter on cohesion. Carol Schreiner and Dorritt Weiss merit special thanks for the hours they spent typing the manuscript. We are grateful to Kathleen Adams Springer who unselfishly donated her time to read the galley proofs. We thankfully acknowledge the contributions of the Road-House staff as well as the staffs of crisis calling/hotline centers across the country, upon whose experience this book is based.

U.D.
E.H.R.
J.T.

To Ursula,

We thank you for sharing your idea for this book with us and for your constant harassment in getting it completed.

Janet and Ed

CONTENTS

CRISIS CENTER/HOTLINE

I

VOLUNTEERS: WHO ARE THEY?

DAVID W. SMART

URING the last decade, the service professions have under-
gone a number of changes as they have sought to improve
mental health services. As greater and greater demands have been
placed upon professional mental health workers, it has become apparent that new procedures must be developed in order to accomodate
the flood of people seeking help. One result of the increased demand
for professional services has been the redefining of the roles of
various mental health workers and the sharing of more and more
responsibilities with laymen. This has given rise to a more broadly
based community mental health movement in which concerned laymen now share responsibilities for education, prevention, and treatment of mental health problems. Professionals have more frequently
been cast in the roles of consultants and trainers as they have attempted to organize and coordinate a vast reservoir of laymen who are
motivated to expand and improve the services offered. Bennett (1966)
stated:

> A broad spectrum of professional activities is emerging, generally char-
> acterized as community mental health. It involves active participation
> in community affairs on the part of mental health personnel, preventive
> intervention at the community level, and collaboration with responsible
> laymen in reducing community tensions. Consultant services are being
> developed for working with and through other professional groups in
> support of mental health. The community itself is being taught to col-
> laborate in creating health-giving environments (p. 1).

Nowhere has this trend been more evident than in the rapid
growth of the number of telephone emergency service centers that
have sprung up across the country. These campus and community
"rap lines" or "hot lines" draw almost exclusively upon volunteers
to staff them.

A survey conducted by Banning and Aulepp (1971) gives some idea of the number of these services now in existence. This survey gathered data about mental health services provided by 117 institutions of higher education in the 13 Western states and, among other things, found that a substantial number offer a telephone emergency service. Table I-I shows the number and percentage of schools of various sizes which reported such service available.

The same report also indicated the existence of an additional 20 crisis programs, organized and administered by students, which were not centered around the use of the telephone.

Who are these "responsible" lay mental health workers to whom Bennett refers and to whom falls the task of staffing these telephone services? Are they indeed responsible? These are important questions which must be answered if the helping professions are to rely more and more heavily upon volunteer and paraprofessional workers. Otherwise the widespread use of what amounts to ill-trained and unprepared laymen may result in the lowering of professional standards, as appears to be the concern of many.

Some controversy exists as to the effectiveness of lay counselors, but the majority of those who have adddressed themselves to this topic have reported favorable results. Carkhuff, who has been quite outspoken in his support of the use of lay counselors, asserted the following: "The lay person's motivation to help appears more simple and direct, unconfounded by needs to find position, status, prestige, money, and perhaps some 'handles' on his own psychological difficulties within the helping role (p. 89)."

Elsewhere, Carkhuff (1968b) has provided a detailed and well-documented comparison of the effectiveness of lay and professional counselors, in which he concluded that lay workers are as effective as the professionals.

TABLE I-I
NUMBER AND PERCENTAGE OF SCHOOLS
WITH TELEPHONE EMERGENCY SERVICE

Enrollment of School	Number	Percentage
Less than 1,000	1	6.7
1000 to 5000	9	17.6
5000 to 10,000	9	42.9
10,000 to 20,000	11	57.9
20,000 or more	7	63.6
Total	37	31.6

A pioneer effort in the training of lay counselors was the program conducted by Rioch *et al.* (1963), in which mature married women were selected for training. The nine candidates selected for this program had a median age of about 40 and were highly educated before beginning the training program. Five of the nine candidates had been in psychotherapy or psychoanalysis for more than two years.

Strikingly similar to those trained by Rioch were the volunteers who staffed the Los Angeles Suicide Prevention Center. Pretzel (1970) described the average or typical LASPC volunteer as (a) a woman; (b) 44 years of age; (c) married with three children; (d) having two years of college education; and interestingly, (e) one who had experienced in her own family background some suicidal behavior or serious mental health problem which required hospitalization. In addition, the typical volunteer had been in therapy for an average of a two-year duration. However, the composite Minnesota Multiphasic Personality Inventory profile of the volunteers revealed little pathology.

Others (Gottesfeld, Rhee, and Parker, 1970; McCarthy and Berman, 1971; McCarthy and Michaud, 1971; Muro, 1970; Pyle and Snyder, 1971) have also indicated successful use of volunteers in a variety of roles. Little, however, has been said about the selection and training procedures which these volunteers have gone through. These procedures appear to vary a great deal with few, if any, widely used guidelines concerning selection and training being applied.

Several writers (Gallagher and Weisbrod, 1970; Heilig *et al.*, 1968; Resnik, 1968; Whittington, 1971) have cautioned against indiscriminate use of paraprofessionals or have provided data which would suggest caution in the use of volunteers. Heilig *et al.*, (1968), in listing the selection criteria for volunteers, went on to report:

> Certain volunteers were avoided. These were especially people looking for a way to gratify their own needs and to push their own individual conceptions of human problems and their solutions. Their investment was frequently in such areas as astrology, hypnotism, spiritualism, numerology, graphology, and others. Often, such persons were emotionally disturbed themselves, rigid, inflexible, and tenuously organized. It was felt that such persons would not serve the agency, they would use it (p. 289).

Of particular interest is Resnik's (1968) study in which he reported a high percentage of neurotic and psychotic lay persons volunteering for work with an anti-suicide telephone service. Based on results from a psychiatric interview, and a battery of tests including the MMPI, House-Tree-Person Drawings, and a sentence-completion test, 22 volunteers (13 women and 9 men) were judged to be normal, neurotic, or psychotic. While seven workers (32%) were considered normal, nine (41%) were judged neurotic and six (27%) psychotic! Resnik did not appear to find this surprising, since he considered the ranks of mental health workers to be replete with those who have consciously and unconsciously sought solutions to personal problems and assumed that such persons may be drawn to community volunteer programs. His study also reported that the disturbed individuals, particularly the psychotics, tended to drop out earlier, work less and respond less adequately when on phone duty.

VOLUNTEERS AT THE UNIVERSITY OF NORTHERN COLORADO AND COLORADO STATE UNIVERSITY

This section describes some characteristics of students who volunteered to staff the emergency telephone service at the University of Northern Colorado. Some comparisons with volunteers of the Colorado State University telephone service and a control group of UNC students are also presented.

The Inception of "Somebody Loves You Baby" Phone Service

A rap line was begun on the UNC campus in January, 1970, and has continued to operate until the present. The impetus for beginning the service was given by Reverend William C. Bingham, the Episcopal chaplain at the university. Various campus agencies including the Counseling Center and the Health Service collaborated in providing physical facilities and consultation services as the rap line was developed. The name "Somebody Loves You Baby" was chosen for the service.

Recruiting Volunteers

Initially few, if any, selection criteria were applied to those who expressed a willingness to work on the phones. Students found out about the service informally by word of mouth and by articles in the campus and local newspapers. Students from a variety of majors and all class levels of the university responded and were included in the initial group of volunteers.

As this body of volunteers began to assemble and grow, the need was felt to gather some kind of data which would possibly assist in forming future selection criteria, or at least give some description of the types of persons who had volunteered. Consequently, the California Psychological Inventory was chosen as an instrument to be administered to all volunteers. Later they were also given the Self Assessment of Attitudes Toward Suicide scale. Some of those who had shown a passing interest as volunteers but dropped out before working on the phones did not take the CPI or Self Assessment of Attitudes Toward Suicide scale.

The California Psychological Inventory (CPI)

This instrument is an objective personality test which yields scores on 18 different scales. It's author (Gough, 1964) intended that the CPI be used primarily with "normal" (nonpsychiatrically disturbed) individuals in such settings as schools, colleges, business, and industry and in counseling agencies whose clientele is not extremely disturbed. The 18 CPI scales are intended to cover various facets of interpersonal functioning and social interaction. The names of the scales were chosen to describe the various kinds of behavior they were designed to reflect. While the CPI manual and its list of bibliographic references present data which help establish the test's validity, no test can be said to be completely validated and unfailingly accurate. The CPI is no exception. It has also been criticized for having so many scales, some of which apparently overlap in what they measure. The names of the scales are listed in Table I-IV along with the scores obtained by the subjects of the study.

The Experimental and Control Groups

In order to make the CPI scores of the UNC and CSU volunteers more meaningful, another UNC group was chosen for the purpose of comparison. The following several paragraphs will present descriptive material on these three groups so that some comparisons between these groups can be made.

The UNC volunteers numbered 91, of whom 40 were men and 51 women. It is not particularly surprising that the women outnumbered the men, since women outnumber men at UNC in a ratio of about five to four. The men had a mean age of 21.32 and the women's

TABLE I-II
MAJORS OF UNC TELEPHONE SERVICE VOLUNTEERS

Major	Frequency	Major	Frequency
Psychology	19	Music	2
Elementary education	12	Biology	2
Special education	9	Mathematics	2
Social science	6	Health education	1
Sociology	4	Science education	1
Vocational rehabilitation	3	Geography	1
Recreation	2	Spanish	1
English	6	History	1
Business	3	Anthropology	1
Art	2	Undecided	11
Nursing	2		

mean age was 21.22. As Table I-II shows, they represented a variety of academic majors.

The relatively high number of education majors among the volunteers reflects the fact that UNC is largely a teacher preparation institution and itself has a high proportion of education majors. Noteworthy also is the large number of psychology majors to be found among the volunteers. Since its inception, the phone service has continued to draw a relatively high proportion of psychology students as volunteers.

The control group consisted of 94 UNC students who were randomly chosen from a group of 351 Professional Teacher Education (PTE) candidates. Since UNC is an institution which has been primarily a school for the preparation of teachers, large numbers of its students acquire teacher certification. During the 1970-71 school year, 72 percent of the 1745 students receiving bachelors degrees also received teaching certificates, these representing a very sizeable proportion of the UNC student body. Professional Teacher Education status is reserved for upperclassmen who have progressed satisfactorily through approximately two years of undergraduate work and who have been screened by means of a psychological inventory. The control group was randomly chosen from the 351 students who presented themselves for the psychological screening test session during the fall quarter of 1971. The 94 students selected for the control group were mostly sophomores and juniors, with the men reporting a mean age of 22.33 years and the women a mean age of 20.75. They represented many different academic majors, as can be seen in Table I-III.

Colorado State University students established a telephone emergency service in 1970, which has been in continuous operation since

TABLE I-III
MAJORS OF PROFESSIONAL TEACHER EDUCATION CANDIDATES

Major	Frequency	Major	Frequency
Elementary education	29	Earth science	1
Special education	15	History	1
Physical education	10	Chemistry	1
Business education	6	Biology	1
Psychology	6	Mathematics	1
Deaf education	4	English	1
Home economics	4	Art	1
Music	5	Speech pathology	1
Fine arts	2	Spanish	1
Social science	2	French	1
Theatre arts	1		

that time. This service, RoadHouse, is staffed entirely by university students but has access to an advisory board of professional counselors who are involved in selection and training procedures. At first, however, RoadHouse volunteers were self-selected in that all interested students who applied were accepted into the training program with no selection criteria being applied other than occasional guidance from advisors. The volunteers included in this study were recruited in this manner before the present selection and training procedures were instituted. The CPI was administered to this sample of students which included 26 women and 18 men from a variety of areas of study who had mean ages of 19.96 and 21.67 years respectively.* A more complete description of the current operating procedures of RoadHouse are given in this volume in the chapters dealing with selection and training of volunteers.

The *t* test of means was applied to the CPI scores of the men and women of all three groups (UNC volunteers, CSU volunteers, PTE candidates) to test for differences between the groups on the various CPI scales. Table I-IV presents means and standard deviations and Table I-V presents the statistical comparisons of these groups.

Discussion of CPI Results

As can be seen from the statistical comparisons of the UNC and CSU volunteers and the PTE candidates, some differences do emerge. However, these differences were not found when the UNC and CSU groups were compared to the national norm groups reported in the

---

*I gratefully acknowledge the generous assistance of Lucinda Thomas who provided the CPI scores of the CSU volunteers.

TABLE I-IV
MEANS AND STANDARD DEVIATIONS OF THREE GROUPS ON CPI SCALES

CPI Scales	UNC Volunteers				CSU Volunteers				PTE Candidates			
	Men N=40		Women N=51		Men N=18		Women N=25		Men N=30		Women N=64	
	M	SD	M	SD	M	SD	M	SD	M	SD	M	SD
Dominance	27.47	6.56	30.25	4.83	31.39	4.69	29.92	5.84	30.00	5.70	27.77	5.69
Capacity for status	19.32	3.90	21.47	3.23	21.68	3.20	21.72	4.06	20.73	3.73	19.41	3.87
Sociability	22.65	4.50	25.83	4.42	26.79	4.88	26.12	4.33	26.98	3.67	24.77	4.60
Social presence	37.05	6.11	39.76	5.45	42.61	4.15	40.60	5.54	39.57	4.28	36.48	6.06
Self-acceptance	22.32	3.44	23.63	3.04	24.78	3.86	24.36	3.89	23.20	3.17	22.19	3.58
Sense of well-being	33.80	6.33	35.75	4.34	36.22	5.04	35.36	3.97	39.07	3.59	37.12	4.43
Responsibility	25.15	4.77	29.41	3.91	26.44	4.85	28.56	3.98	29.17	5.18	30.88	4.45
Socialization	30.90	6.09	34.59	5.63	33.00	5.16	34.52	4.53	36.23	3.60	39.42	5.07
Self-control	24.02	6.63	27.02	7.06	27.33	5.09	24.76	6.48	38.17	7.68	30.70	6.45
Tolerance	20.55	5.31	23.06	3.46	24.22	3.77	22.92	3.64	23.60	4.21	23.42	4.27
Good impression	15.17	4.82	17.96	5.18	16.83	4.88	15.08	5.31	17.67	5.90	18.22	5.96
Communality	23.67	3.08	25.20	2.27	24.94	2.10	24.84	2.43	26.00	1.82	26.17	1.86
Achievement via conformance	23.88	4.49	26.92	4.62	26.44	5.74	25.12	3.44	27.03	5.20	28.44	4.29
Achievement via independence	21.52	4.04	22.65	3.23	23.67	2.58	22.36	3.88	19.90	4.45	21.16	3.79
Intellectual efficiency	26.67	5.77	40.10	4.26	41.78	3.92	39.76	4.95	40.50	4.30	39.80	4.16
Psychological mindedness	12.07	2.70	12.47	2.61	14.17	2.20	12.44	2.68	12.07	2.98	11.45	2.35
Flexibility	14.17	3.54	14.06	3.29	14.67	3.22	14.88	2.71	11.87	3.13	11.08	3.67
Femininity	18.82	3.41	22.71	3.16	17.22	3.90	22.56	3.02	14.93	3.09	23.69	2.94

TABLE I-V

SIGNIFICANCE OF RESULTS IN GROUP COMPARISONS

CPI Scales	Men			Women		
	UNC Volunteers and PTE	CSU Volunteers and PTE	UNC Volunteers and CSU Volunteers	UNC Volunteers and PTE	CSU Volunteers and PTE	UNC Volunteers and CSU Volunteers
	t test	t test	t test	t test	t test	t test
Dominance	1.68	.82	2.19*	2.49*	1.59	.26
Capacity for status	1.52	.88	2.28*	3.06†	2.50*	.29
Sociability	4.29†	.15	3.15†	1.25	1.26	.28
Social presence	1.93	2.41*	3.51†	3.01*	2.95†	.62
Self-acceptance	1.09	1.54	2.42*	2.29*	2.51*	.90
Sense of well-being	4.09†	2.28*	1.43	1.67	1.74	.37
Responsibility	3.36†	1.80	.95	1.85	2.27*	.89
Socialization	4.27‡	2.56*	1.27	4.84‡	4.22‡	.05
Self-control	2.51*	.41	1.88	2.92*	3.90‡	1.35
Tolerance	2.59*	.51	2.64*	.49	.52	.16
Good impression	1.94	.50	1.21	.24	2.30*	2.26*
Communality	3.67‡	1.84	1.58	2.54	2.78†	.63
Achievement via conformance	2.72†	.36	1.84	1.82	3.45‡	1.73
Achievement via independence	1.59	3.25†	2.05*	2.24*	1.34	.34
Intellectual efficiency	3.05†	1.03	3.40†	.38	.04	.31
Psychological mindedness	.01	2.59*	2.88†	2.20*	1.71	.05
Flexibility	2.83†	2.97†	.50	4.53‡	4.70‡	1.08
Femininity	4.91‡	2.25*	1.58	1.72	1.62	.19

*Significant at .05 level
†Significant at .01 level
‡Significant at .001 level

CPI manual. This would suggest that there may indeed be some identifiable differences between the local groups, but that these differences are not apparent when the local groups are compared to the large national norm sample.

However, considering the local group comparisons, one rather consistent difference between both groups of phone volunteers and the control group is evident—the higher Flexibility score of the volunteers. All phone volunteer groups (UNC and CSU men and women) scored higher on the Flexibility scale than did control group men or women. This would suggest that the phone volunteers were more flexible and adaptable in their thinking and social behavior and less rigid and deferential to authority and tradition than the PTE candidates.

Another difference between the volunteer and control group can be seen on the Socialization scale. In this case all volunteer groups were lower on the socialization scale than was the control group. This would suggest a tendency for these lay mental health counselors to behave with less maturity, integrity and rectitude, and to be less conscientious and responsible than their fellow students who are seeking teacher certification.

Also noted was the tendency for telephone volunteers to be more autonomous and independent rather than conforming in their mode of achievement as compared to the PTE group. That is, volunteers would be more likely to achieve in settings in which autonomy and independence are prized rather than in settings where conformity and cooperation are expected.

Another tendency emerged from the testing data which would suggest that the volunteers are apt to be less self-controlled than the prospective teachers. Three of the four subgroups of phone workers (UNC men, UNC women, and CSU women) obtained significantly lower scores on the Self-control scale than did the PTE men or women. Accordingly, phone workers would tend to manifest less self-regulation and more impulsivity than the control group.

One additional tendency is suggested by the data—the tendency for the male volunteers to possess certain feminine characteristics when compared to the PTE candidates. The higher scores on the Femininity scale are indicative of the male phone workers being more appreciative, patient, helpful, gentle, and moderate versus their education counterparts who would be seen as being more hard-headed, active, blunt and direct. This brings to mind Farson's (1954) article entitled, "The Counselor is a Woman," in which he stresses the point that the role of the counselor is often that of being sensitive, gentle, and helpful in a rather passive way. The male phone volunteers would appear to fit that description.

As noted earlier, however, these above-mentioned differences between the experimental and control groups were not found when statistical comparisons to the national norm groups were made. This is due, in part, to the large difference in sample size between the two experimental groups and the national norm group. So much of the variance in the distribution of scores is contributed by the large norm group, that differences between the groups are masked.

The Self Assessment of Attitudes Toward Suicide Scale

An additional evaluation of the UNC phone volunteers was carried out about one year after the phone service had been in operation. This evaluation was conducted with the volunteers who were in training at that particular time and did not include some of the more experienced workers who had already been trained. The instrument which was used for this evaluation was the Self Assessment of Attitudes Toward Suicide scale, a 17-item instrument which was constructed by Klainer, Murray, and Beller, Inc., a health systems consulting firm, in consultation with the Center for Studies of Suicide Prevention of the National Institute of Mental Health. The development of this instrument is still in its experimental stage, although it has been used in evaluating a pilot curriculum study in suicidology which is being developed by the Center for Studies of Suicide Prevention. The self-assessment instrument is based upon the method of summated ratings on a seven-point scale which ranges from "strongly agree" to "strongly disagree." The content of the items runs from general questions about one's attitude toward suicide to items which deal with what one would do if confronted with a person who was contemplating suicide.

The UNC Volunteer Group and the Control Group

As mentioned above, the volunteer group which took the attitude assessment instrument did not include some of those who had volunteered and worked on the phones the previous year as did the group which took the CPI. The UNC volunteers who took the suicide attitude test numbered 60 (28 men and 32 women), and came from a variety of majors as seen in Table I-VI.

TABLE I-VI
MAJORS OF UNC VOLUNTEERS IN ATTITUDES TOWARD SUICIDE
SAMPLE

Major	Frequency	Major	Frequency
Psychology	18	Biology	1
Elementary education	6	Music	1
Special education	5	Mathematics	1
Sociology	4	Nursing	1
Social science	3	Science education	1
Vocational rehabilitation	3	Health education	1
Behavioral science	2	Fine arts	1
Business	2	Geography	1
English	2	Undecided	5
Recreation	2		

These volunteers came from all levels of university as follows: 11 freshmen, 23 sophomores, 15 juniors, seven seniors and four graduate students.

At the same time that the phone volunteers took the attitude assessment scale, a random sample of 100 UNC students was chosen to provide a comparison group on the attitude scale. These randomly chosen students were sent a copy of the assessment inventory together with instructions on how to fill it out. They were requested to take the inventory and return it in the enclosed envelope. A return of 71 was obtained from the sample of 100.

The 71 students (29 men and 40 women) of this control group came from all levels of the university in the following numbers: 12 freshmen, 18 sophomores, 26 juniors, 11 seniors and four graduate students. Table I-VII presents an analysis of the various majors of this group.

TABLE I-VII
MAJORS OF UNC ATTITUDES TOWARD SUICIDE CONTROL GROUP

Major	Frequency	Major	Frequency
Elementary education	12	Vocational education	1
Business	10	Speech pathology	1
Special education	8	Physical education	1
Nursing	5	Speech	1
Psychology	5	Pre-medicine	1
Sociology	3	Chemistry	1
English	3	Art	1
Fine arts	3	Home economics	1
Mathematics	3	Economics	1
Social science	2	Recreation	1
Music	2	Undecided	3
Industrial arts	2		

The greatest difference between the distribution of majors of the volunteers and the control group is that there are considerably fewer psychology majors in the control group.

The *t* test of means was applied to the scores of the attitude assessment scale to test for differences between the groups. Table I-VIII presents the means, standard deviations, and *t* values for both groups.

As can be seen from Table I-VIII, significant differences between the volunteers and the control group were obtained on items 10, 13 and 17. Because only three test items proved to differ significantly between the two groups, it can be inferred that the groups are really quite similar in their attitudes toward suicide. One would expect

TABLE I-VIII
COMPARISON OF SCORES ON SELF-ASSESSMENT OF
ATTITUDES TOWARD SUICIDE SCALE

Scale Item	UNC Volunteers N=60		UNC Control Group N=71		
	M	SD	M	SD	t
1	4.82	1.90	4.68	1.95	.42
2	4.62	2.08	4.46	2.03	.42
3	5.78	1.48	5.30	1.80	1.67
4	2.00	1.18	2.28	1.62	1.12
5	4.10	1.75	4.66	1.94	1.72
6	4.40	1.93	4.18	2.15	.60
7	2.35	1.54	2.10	1.46	1.28
8	5.80	1.35	5.58	1.53	.86
9	1.83	1.19	1.99	1.43	.65
10	3.18	1.50	3.90	1.67	2.56*
11	3.40	1.81	2.90	1.77	1.59
12	2.75	1.88	2.37	1.64	1.25
13	3.57	1.76	4.28	1.61	2.42*
14	2.50	1.61	2.84	1.77	1.16
15	1.81	1.14	1.84	1.25	.13
16	2.75	1.70	3.13	1.93	1.17
17	2.98	1.84	4.13	2.13	3.26†

*Significant at .05 level
†Significant at .01 level

about one item out of 20 to differ significantly at the .05 level simply because of chance variations. Since only three test items indicate differences of opinion on this particular scale with these two groups, little besides chance variation appears to be operating. However, two of the differing items are concerned with how one would react to a person who is contemplating suicide. The responses of the volunteer group suggest a tendency to feel more comfortable in working with such an individual. This must, however, be taken as a tentative interpretation of these results.

Academic Ability of Volunteers

American College Testing Program scores are required of UNC students before they are admitted to the university. However, some exceptions are made and it is possible to transfer to UNC without having taken the ACT. In searching the records of UNC phone volunteers, it was found that ACT scores were available for 79 students, or 84 percent of the 94 volunteers who were tested with the CPI. Table I-IX gives a comparison of ACT composite scores of these 79 volunteers and the UNC freshman class of 1969.

No significant difference between the volunteers and the UNC

TABLE I-IX
COMPARISON OF ACT COMPOSITE SCORES

Volunteers N=79		Freshmen N=1588		
M	SD	M	SD	t
20.7	5.8	21.4	3.9	1.03

freshmen who entered in 1969 was found in this comparison of ACT composite scores. This would indicate that there is no difference in academic ability between the two groups.

CONCLUSIONS

The trend toward increased involvement of lay persons in mental health services is likely to continue and will probably accelerate. Studies have been reported which suggest that lay mental health counselors can be effectively employed in a wide variety of helping roles. However, there is also evidence to suggest that not all who volunteer to serve in a helping capacity are qualified. Certainly some are better suited to become engaged in such activities than are others. It would appear that at the present time greater care must be exercised in selecting and training volunteer mental health workers. In many instances, selection criteria appear to be applied in rather haphazard fashion, if applied at all.

The results of the present study, however, are viewed as being encouraging in that no great differences or deficiencies were evident in the samples of volunteer phone workers described. There is some evidence to suggest that the volunteers were quite flexible, open individuals, a characteristic often found in professional mental health workers of various disciplines. On the other hand, there appeared to be a tendency for volunteers to be less socialized and more impulsive than may be ideal, but in general, no striking deficiencies were noted. Also, an instrument designed to assess attitudes toward suicide revealed few, if any, differences between volunteer phone workers and a control group. In addition, no differences in academic ability between volunteers and a comparison group of university freshmen were found.

REFERENCES

Banning, J. H. and Aulepp, L.: Program activities and student utilization of campus mental health facilities in the west. *Western Interstate Commission on Higher Education,* 1971, No. 3.

Bennett, C. (Ed.): *Community Psychology*. Boston, Boston University, 1966.

Carkhuff, R. R.: Lay mental health counseling: prospects and problems. *Journal of Counseling Psychology, 15:*117-126, 1968.

Farson, R. E.: The counselor is a woman. *Journal of Counseling Psychology, 1:*221-223, 1954.

Gallagher, P. J. and Weisbrod, K. C.: The counseling psychologist. In Gallagher, P. J. Demos, G. D. (Eds.): *The Counseling Center in Higher Education* Springfield, Thomas, 1970.

Gough, H. G.: *California Psychological Inventory Manual*. Palo Alto, Consulting Psychology Press, Inc., 1964.

Gottesfeld, H., Rhee, C. and Parker, G.: A study of the role of paraprofessionals in community mental health. *Community Mental Health Journal, 6:*285-291, 1970.

Heilig, S. M. *et al:* The role of nonprofessional volunteers in a suicide prevention center. *Community Mental Health Journal, 4:*287-295, 1968.

McCarthy, B. W. and Berman, A. L.: The development of a student-operated crisis center. *Personnel and Guidance Journal, 49:*523-528, 1971.

McCarthy, B. W. and Michaud, P. A.: Companions: an adjunct to counseling. *Personnel and Guidance Journal, 49:*839-841, 1971.

Muro, J. J.: Community volunteers: a new thrust for guidance. *Personnel and Guidance Journal, 49:*137-141, 1970.

Pretzel, P. W.: The volunteer clinical worker at the suicide prevention center. *Bulletin of Suicidology, 6:*27-34, 1970.

Pyle, R. R. and Snyder, F. A.: Students as paraprofessional counselors at community colleges. *Journal of College Student Personnel, 12:*259-263, 1971.

Resnik, H. L. P.: A community anti-suicide organization: the friends of Dade County, Florida. In Resnik, H. L. P. (Ed.): *Suicidal Behaviors Diagnosis and Management*. Boston, Little Brown and Company, 1968.

Rioch, Margaret *et al.:* National institute of mental mealth pilot study in training mental health counselors. *American Journal of Orthopsychiatry, 33:* 678-689, 1963.

Whittington, H. G.: Crisis centers—collegiate and community. Paper presented at the Fifth Annual Workshop for Emotional Problems of College Students, University of Northern Colorado, Greeley, Colorado, 1971.

II

SELECTION: WHO CAN BE HELPFUL?

Ursula Delworth

THE staff of any crisis center is the key to its success. Without effective helpers all other ingredients will be useless in providing a viable service.

Effective staff are produced through two essential developments: selection and training. Training without proper selection is usually inefficient and can also be pointless and ineffective in the long run.

Thus far, crisis centers have rarely employed any standard procedures in selecting their volunteers. Often, there is a screening interview to weed out the obviously unstable. Many centers report that they accept most applicants, then observe them closely during training and/or the initial weeks of service to determine if they should continue with the center.

In a number of programs, new workers are assigned more clerically oriented tasks until the staff can decide whether they should be allowed to give direct service.

These procedures make some sense when the center is new or very few persons are applying to be volunteers. However, more efficient and effective selection procedures become necessary when more persons than can be accommodated wish to join the staff. This is a situation which occurs in most centers sooner or later.

There is another issue involved here as well, which is relevant even to centers which are just opening and have few potential staff members from whom to select. Research clearly shows (Eysenck, 1952; Bergin, 1966) that intended "help" can have deteriorating or negative effects upon the person seeking help. Therefore, it seems vital to utilize selection procedures in order to train only those who show promise of being truly helpful to others.

DEFINING THE JOB

The first crucial question is, "What are these volunteers going to do?" A clear definition of the job is necessary before it is possible to set up selection criteria.

The primary step is to be specific about services to be offered by the center. Once this is clear, a job description outlining the duties and levels of functioning can be written.

The following outline can serve to delineate relevant dimensions of responsibility.

A. Interpersonal
    1. Is the volunteer at the center totally self-reliant? Is there a back-up person on call?
    2. Does the volunteer do actual counseling, or is the service providing listening and referral only?
    3. Is the volunteer expected to have specific skills, such as talking a person "down" from a bad trip?
B. Administration
    1. What records does the volunteer keep?
    2. What responsibilities for center operation does he assume?
C. Information
    1. Does the volunteer need to know a great deal of information regarding the resources available to clients of the center, or are these resources so limited that he need learn only a few key ones?
    2. Is the volunteer expected to have much information in specific areas (drugs, draft, abortion, etc.)? If so, which ones?
D. Type of Service
    1. If the service is phone only, what specific telephone skills does the volunteer need?
    2. If the service is a walk-in, what additional skills are considered important?

The job description should be as specific as possible regarding these dimensions, and should also rank-order the qualifications as much as possible. For example, if record keeping is important but not crucial, this skill might be listed rather low on the priority list.

SELECTION SKILLS

It is critical next to determine which of these skills are abilities the prospective volunteer must possess at the time of application and which can be taught later. Generally, well-established centers in metropolitan areas have the largest pool from which to choose their volunteers and thus can be more selective. That is, they can accept only those who already possess most of the qualifications necessary for the job. They can then cut down on training time and/or concentrate during that time on specific skills which the applicants do not already possess.

Smaller centers often find that they have fewer applicants, and that most of these possess limited skills in the areas outlined in the job description. At that point, a decision must be made regarding which qualifications are most important for selection. Others can be built into the training program later.

If specific information or mechanical skills are part of the necessary qualifications, a straightforward question-and-answer device can be used. This can be verbal, written, or demonstrated, as in the case of a skill like typing.

A number of centers are more concerned with qualifications in the interpersonal area. They want both to screen out "sick" applicants, and select those who indicate the most potential for becoming "helping persons." It is much more difficult to devise selection procedures in this area.

Often direct questions concerning an applicant's motivation is helpful here. Interviewers can look for both a desire on the part of the applicant to be of aid to others, as well as to develop skills for himself. In our experience, these goals appear together in the effective volunteer. He can pay attention both to his needs and those of others. Questions also often can determine whether the prospective volunteer is both willing and able to leave his own problems outside the door when he comes to work in the center. Most services do not expect (nor especially want) their volunteers to be problem-free, but they do expect that the volunteer can be tuned in to others while he is on duty.

Some centers have utilized personality tests or inventories for assessment of interpersonal functioning. When interpreted by a professional familiar with the test, these measures can yield information on pathology, or nonhealthful functioning. This way, the least healthy or stable applicants can be eliminated.

However, no personality traits per se as measured by these devices have been found to be generally more indicative of "helpers" vs "non-helpers." These tests are a very indirect method, subject to much interpretation, and in general we would not recommend their use. There are more direct ways to tune in on a person's level of functioning, usually with less threat to the individual.

HELPFUL DEVELOPMENTS

Helpful answers to the question of assessment of interpersonal functioning are being provided by two recent developments in the field of human service.

The first of these is the work of the New Careers movement (Pearl and Riessman, 1965; McLennon *et al.*, 1966; Riessman and Popper, 1968), which offers employment and concurrent education as a way out of poverty. New Careers developers clearly articulate the necessity for a close tie between selection procedures and the job to be done. Training is perceived as primarily the in-service type (as it is in many crisis centers), so that New Careerists begin to function on the job with little pre-service training. Therefore, it is important to select those with some already developed "people skills."

Among the techniques developed has been an extensive use of role playing in a near-realistic situation. In some cases, actual recipients of the agency's service are hired to take part in simulated interview experiences, and then give feedback to the agency regarding the performance of the applicant. A variation on this for telephone centers involves the use of a telephone interview of the prospective applicant, which may involve having him respond to a simulated crisis situation. These techniques emphasize the strengths of many helpers who are better at *doing* than at talking about *how* to do it.

Riessman (1967) also advocates a group interview procedure in which one or more interviewers meet with several applicants for New Careers positions. This is a way of observing how potential volunteers interact with peers rather than just with agency representatives.

The second promising development is the work of Robert Carkhuff (1969). He has defined as a selection principle the idea that the best index of whether a person will be helpful to another is his *current* functioning as a helping person. He utilizes scales of discrimination and communication in selecting those who will receive further training. The scales are based on his research with the facilitative and action-oriented dimensions relevant in the helping process. These include such areas as *empathy* (understanding), *respect* and *confrontation*. Carkhuff advocates the selection of those who are currently rated as "most helpful" on the scales, since these persons have the most potential for development. (This assumes trainers who are functioning at still higher levels than the trainees, however.)

Each of Carkhuff's scales consists of the same sixteen helpee excerpts, that is, brief statements made by persons seeking aid. They deal with a variety of content and feeling areas. In the communication index, the helper formulates his own response to the excerpt. With the discrimination index, four possible responses are given and the applicant is asked to rate each on a scale from one to five. The applicant is thus attempting to discriminate between good and poor responses. Brief directions regarding how to rate the responses are included.

Although Carkhuff's excerpts are a good place to start, centers are encouraged to develop their own. These will be based on the common problems which are presented by users of the agency's service and may seem more relevant to applicants. For example, a university center will utilize excerpts or situations common to the campus.

The excerpts can be presented in written, audio, or audiovisual form. It makes sense to employ the modality in which the helping service will be offered, if at all possible. For example, an audio presentation is appropriate for a phone service. Generally, the responses will have to be written, unless there is a setup available in which persons can respond both independently and simultaneously. Some college language labs are equipped to provide for this.

Research suggests that discrimination is a necessary but not sufficient condition for good communication. That is, good communicators are also good discriminators, but not every person who does well on discrimination will be a helpful communicator. Since crisis centers are in the business of helping others through facilitative communication, it is much more important to concentrate on this aspect during selection.

One problem here is that a communication scale demands that someone rate the responses that the prospective helper makes to the excerpt. Persons have to be carefully trained to do this. Also, this rating procedure takes a good deal of time, especially in cases in which there are many applicants.

Sometimes, therefore, it may make sense to utilize the discrimination index, at least as a preliminary screening device. This can be easily scored, using Carkhuff's book or by referring to a scale developed at the center itself. A discrimination index developed for use in selection of volunteers for RoadHouse, Colorado State University's crisis center, is presented at the end of the chapter. It was developed by six student trainers. This scale can best be utilized in conjunction with a more thorough understanding of the core dimensions of the helping relationship, as presented by Carkhuff. Although in agreement with his dimensions, we found Carkhuff's scale to have limited value and appeal in a university crisis center situation. Thus, we developed our own along similiar lines, and hopefully using the same rating methods. Our research indicates that students score about the same on both indexes, but prefer the excerpts developed by Road-House.

The communication scales, besides being a selection device, serve as an excellent pre-training check. Applicants can be asked to "tune in" to themselves as they make their responses, and note those content and feeling areas that make them particularly anxious. These are areas that they can then pay special attention to during the training process.

Carkhuff also suggests the use of a training analogue, that is, a brief training session, as part of the selection process. He asserts that those who can utilize a small amount of training effectively will be best able to utilize an extended training experience.

In such an analogue, for example, applicants might spend two hours learning and practicing more emphatic responses or improving listening skills. Those who catch on most quickly and seem to be able to use the skill best are selected. This is an especially important procedure when pre-service training will be limited. It is vital in this case to select those who can learn quickly.

TRAINERS

Selection of trainers should be taken at least as seriously as the selection of volunteers. Only those who are highly effective in a specific area should be allowed to train others in that area. This means, minimally, that the trainer should score higher or be rated more highly than applicants on any indexes used. He must be more knowledgeable about drugs than the volunteers he instructs. He must be more effective as a helper than those he is guiding toward becoming helpful persons.

SUMMARY

In summary, it is possible to articulate several principles of good selection.

1. Outline the requirements for effective staff operation at your center.
2. Decide which of these requirements the applicant must possess when he applies, and which can be covered in training.
3. Develop selection procedures which will tell you if the applicant has the required skills, and to what degree.
4. Select trainers who are more skilled than the volunteers in the areas in which they will be responsible for training.

Remember that current functioning is the best predictor of how a person will function as a volunteer. In all cases, give the prospective volunteer as much chance as possible to show you what he can do, how he presently operates. Look only at those dimensions that are relevant to the kind of service you operate. Adherance to these principles can save a good deal of frustration, extended training, and can result in the offering of a more effective service by volunteers.

CRISIS CENTER DISCRIMINATION INDEX

Introduction

The Index was developed by L. E. Peterson, Leigh W. Allen, Janet Taub, Marta L. Hedde, Janet E. Geis, and Kathleen Adams Springer (RoadHouse staff) working with the author of this chapter.

Table II-I gives the expert rating against which a center using the scale can validate responses. First find the difference between the numerical rating given to each response in the table and the rating given by the person to whom you are administering the scale. Add the differences for each person. The scores can then be used as desired. We have tended not to select persons with total scores of more than 70 to 75, but data is still preliminary. At least you have some data regarding whether your applicants and trainees can differentiate helpful from unhelpful responses. Some variation from the expert ratings is to be expected even with well-trained and experienced persons.

The level of facilitation and action orientation indicates whether a response is high or low on those dimensions. For a further explanation of the dimensions, refer to Carkhuff.

Instructions

These directions can be read by those taking the Index or can be presented to them orally. We suggest a combination—they can be read by the person administering the Index, and a copy should be given to each person for his own reference.

You will read about (listen to) sixteen persons who are seeking help with a problem. They may not be formal clients but simply people who have sought the help of another person in a time of need.

Following each excerpt by a person seeking help you will read (listen to) four possible responses. These are initial responses which might be made early in the course of the helping relationship. Each of the four responses should be rated according to the continuum below. Rate each response independently of the others.

Rate each response 1.0, 1.5, 2.0, 2.5, 3.0, 3.5, 4.0, 4.5, or 5.0.

1.0 1.5	*2.0 2.5*	*3.0 3.5*	*4.0 4.5*	*5.0*
Is not helpful in recognizing the problem; may hinder communication.	Partial recognition of problem and/or feelings towards it.	Minimally helps the person in recognizing the problem and his feelings towards it.	Significantly helps the person in recognizing the problem and dealing with it.	Optimally aids the person in dealing with his problem.

As you judge the responses, keep in mind that the most highly rated responses are those which the person can use most effectively in his present situation.

Excerpt 1

Helpee: What kind of goddamn school do you have here? Jesus, everywhere I go, if it's not a bunch of faggots and queers swishing around, it's the coons and spics reuniting. What the hell kind of place is this anyway—and I expect a decent answer!

Helper Responses:

1. Wow, it seems to me that you are really frustrated with your relationship to these different groups. And it really upsets you, knowing that you will have to relate to them or perhaps find a group that you can genuinely relate with.

2. It sounds like you were raised in a small town or rural area. "Once a country person, always a country person."

3. This is a place where there are a lot of different minorities and this upsets a lot of people. Maybe we can talk about exactly how these different groups have upset you and what we can do about it.

4. Jesus, it seems that those different groups have really turned you off, and it brings you to question the whole school in general.

Excerpt 2

Helpee: I would like your opinion, given this choice. I purchased a tab of acid from a friend of mine. He said it was very mild, a good one for those who have never tripped before. I have always wanted to try LSD once—I have heard all about the controversies and so I believe I know what I'm getting into. However, I would still like to hear what some other people have to say about it. I've made the transition to a freak almost, the acid is the last stage—so can you tell me what acid is all about?

Helper Responses:

1. Listen, I really think you should consider the physiological effects of acid. They can be detrimental to your psychological health as well.

2. Seems like a difficult choice to make. I can see how you might feel it's part of becoming a freak.

3. I hope that no one saw you purchase the tab.

4. Being a freak is pretty important to you. But I sense some hesitancy or conflict in making your decision.

Excerpt 3

Helpee: I have a problem. It's about this guy. You see, I'm gay and I'm having a love quarrel. John, that's the name of my lover, is more straight than gay. He has recently met this girl who is more exciting than me—so he says anyway. If he continues seeing this girl, it will only mean heartbreak for me. I've never thought about suicide before now, but every day just brings more and more confusion. People say I'm strange, and maybe everybody would be just as happy if I happened to disappear.

Helper Responses:

1. Things are pretty confused right now, but don't you think you could find somebody else? Are you perhaps taking this too seriously?

2. Sounds like you're pretty depressed and confused; you feel very

alone and empty because you feel that your relationship with someone you love is very threatened, and possibly over. It seems to mean the whole world to you. But, are you only living because of John?

3. In any personal relationship there are problems. When these problems arise it's good to talk about them to the person who is involved. Have you talked to John about this?

4. Wow, things are really going bad for you—you're feeling pretty depressed and worthless. The loss or possible loss of someone you really care for can be shattering.

Excerpt 4

Helpee: (sobbing) : I've got a terrible problem and I need some answers pretty quick. If your fiancé was away, like going to another school, and you got pregnant by what you thought was a good friend, how would you tell your fiancé the situation? I mean, I'm getting an abortion, so that's all taken care of, he doesn't ever need to know about it, or anything like that, but I feel I've got a responsibility to tell him about the situation. I think he deserves to know about what went on and what a rat I am, but I don't know how to tell him. I just don't know!

Helper Responses:

1. Does your fiancé know the guy who got you pregnant?

2. If you really want it, go ahead and get the abortion and then tell him about everything. That way, he won't have to worry about that aspect. Then, you can proceed from there.

3. Wow, it sounds like you really are in a fix. If you feel like crying, go ahead. Then you can tell me a little more about the situation and we can see what to do from there. Maybe we can think of some alternatives together that would be suitable and make it a little easier for everyone involved.

4. Wow, you really have yourself in a situation that is so confusing that it's difficult to be rational and think up a solution.

Excerpt 5

Helpee: Your ad said that you were interested in other people's problems, so I'm gonna lay a heavy one on you. I've been dating this black chick for about three months now. There wouldn't be a problem except that I'm white. I've been raised to see no difference between white and black and I believe that I exhibit this point of view myself now as an adult. The problem is with my chick who somehow believes that I should see a difference between us—she is always testing me to see if I have yet become a racial bigot. I'm getting tired of this but I feel something special for this chick. As though matters weren't bad enough, she is now pregnant; I believe it is probably my kid, but there always exists the chance that it could be one of her black brother's. So, here is the problem. Now, what is the answer?

Helper Responses:

1. That's a rough one alright. Sounds like you're really rushed to make up your mind about how you feel toward her.

2. Would it be a whole lot less of a hassle if she were white or you two were married?

3. You're right, it is a heavy one. I can see how you'd feel a conflict within your feelings toward her, and now her pregnancy makes some kind of decision mandatory. Maybe pregnancy is some kind of final test?

4. I can't answer it for you; all I can do is help you consider the alternatives.

Excerpt 6

Helpee: I'm so happy I just don't know what to do. I went out with this guy that I've had my eye on since high school. It was so neat! He acts absolutely in love with me. He didn't say anything about calling again, but I'm sure he will.

Helper Responses:

1. You sound as though you might be wondering if you're not reading too much into this one date.

2. You sound like you had a really good time. It's a good feeling to know that one of your hopes might be realized. I'd like to hear more about how things went on the date.

3. Life can be exciting—full of unexpected happiness. How did this date come about?

4. You feel like a long hoped-for door has been opened, and that makes you very happy. It's really neat to feel that one of your dreams might be realized.

Excerpt 7

Helpee: I am flunking a class and I can't afford to flunk it. The teacher is really understanding, but I just can't grasp the material. She spends all kinds of time with me, but it doesn't seem to do any good. I need the credits *now* in order to graduate. I can't get them later because I'm taking maximum loads all the way until graduation. I've considered really going all out and cheating to get through the class, but I can't really justify it. I've got to have the credits one way or another, but I don't know what to do. What would you do in my case?

Helper Responses:

1. Well, it sounds like you're stuck with the class, like it or not. You sound like you're basically against cheating; but the university has a free tutoring service, there are test files you could look into, or maybe even someone in the class could help you. This way, the material would be presented in a different way and maybe help you to grasp it.

2. Maybe if you talked to the prof again and told her you don't understand the material, she'd slow down more for you.

3. Wow, if I were in your shoes, I'd probably flunk the class.

4. I really agree it's a tight situation to be in. I was in a class once where I had to face the choice of cheating.

Excerpt 8

Helpee: Yeah, um . . . I have this problem, and I don't know what anybody's going to do about it, because it's not the sort of thing that has an answer, but . . . oh, a couple of months ago, I met this guy at the Matterhorn, and—I don't know—we sort of hit it off and so I ended up going to his apartment . . . and . . . oh—we drank a little over there, and smoked a little, and I ended up getting really, really drunk and really stoned, and I ended up going to bed with him . . . and . . . well . . . that was okay, I mean, I didn't ever hear from him after that, and that didn't really bother me, because, well, you know, I was kind of embarrassed about it—I mean, I don't usually do things like that, but —I walked into my discussion group for one of my upper division classes this quarter, and lo and behold, he's a grad student and he's teaching the discussion group. I just about died of embarrassment when I walked in, but—I mean, there's nothing I can do. I haven't been back since . . . I can't drop the class, it's a 400-level class, and I need it to graduate, and it isn't offered any other time this year, and I can't change sections, but I just about . . . I mean, I can't sit through a quarter of having this guy laughing at me up there in front of the class, and perhaps telling all of his friends and frat brothers everything else, and it's just—I mean, it really bothers me, I'm so embarrassed about it. And there seems like there's nothing I can do.

Helper Responses:

1. Seems to me you'd know by now that you can't hop in bed with any-body and have it come out okay.

2. If I were you, I'd go right into his office and talk to him about it. Who knows, maybe he feels the same way.

3. Boy, I bet this would be a tense situation. I can see that you are embarrassed about it.

4. Wow, I can tell this really bothers you. Since you've already eliminated some of the possibilities, what do you think would happen if you talked to him in his office or over a cup of coffee?

Excerpt 9

Helpee: Well, you see, I got this girl pregnant and I'm not going to marry her. I want some information about abortions because I feel a certain responsibility. You see, I don't know if I love her or not and I got to be sure before I start thinking about marrying her—I mean, about marrying anyone.

Helper Responses:

1. I hear you saying that this pregnancy has put you in a trap in which you see abortion as the only way out. Perhaps, though, it has raised some basic questions of whether you really love this girl—and if you think you do, is it only because you feel responsible for her preg-nancy?

2. It seems you're feeling like the walls are closing in fast. This girl's pregnancy has raised the question of responsibility and you want to do the right thing.

3. If the girl is definitely pregnant, then abortion *is* one of the alter-natives. Have you and this girl talked about any of the other alternatives? I feel that you should at least look at all that is open to you before you make your final decision.

4. First, let me ask you, what is your definition of love? The way you look at this situation can be based on just that alone.

Excerpt 10

Helpee: What should I do? My son is taking drugs, I just know he has to be. He has been acting very odd ever since his father and I got the divorce last month. It must be his father's doing. He would do anything to take my boy away from me and that father of his is always up to no good.

Helper Responses:

1. What indications do you have that your son is taking drugs, other than he has been acting strange? How can you be sure that his father has something to do with it? Could anything else, say your divorce and the separation of the family, be making your son act strange?

2. Sounds like you're pretty upset about two problems: first, your son and his recent behavior and second, your ex-husband's influence on your son. What specific examples indicate that your son is taking drugs?

3. It's really a disturbing feeling when you think your son is doing something that might be harmful to him. It's doubly disturbing when you think your ex-husband might be involved.

4. Divorce in a family sometimes causes all sorts of hassles. How long has it been since you and your husband were divorced?

Excerpt 11

Helpee: I'm in sort of a bind— I don't know if you can help me, but, well, I've gotten very interested in my roommate's old fiancé. Since he and I have started to become friends she has been treating me very coolly. We were good friends before she moved in, too. I asked her if it bothered her, but she says *no*. I don't think she has the right to tell me who to see, but I don't want to jeopardize our friendship.

Helper Responses:

1. So you want to continue seeing the guy but don't want your relationship with your roommate to suffer?

2. Have you really talked to your roommate in depth about this?

3. I can see the conflict. If you and your roommate are really being truthful with each other, maybe the problem isn't the fact that you are dating the guy, but how tactfully you handle the situation.

4. She sounds like she is really a sore loser.

Excerpt 12

Helpee: I guess you don't deal in this area, but I couldn't think of anybody else to call. I live in ——Hall and I have been here a quarter. My roommate and I have gone on a diet together. She is built like Racquel Welch but I've got about 50 pounds to go. She's always getting me dates with gorgeous boys, but they never call back. I want to meet a nice boy; I guess one who doesn't mind fat.

Helper Responses:

1. It's good that you are working to look your best. But it sounds like you're hurt because guys don't take time to get to know *you,* to look beyond the surface.

2. Could you tell me how much you weigh and how tall you are?

3. Have you tried Weight Watchers? They have an excellent, healthy diet program that's practically foolproof.

4. It sounds like you realize it will take a while to get your weight down, but you want to have fun and date while you're doing it.

Excerpt 13

Helpee: I want to quit school; I'm tired of being broke and having a rundown car and a crappy apartment. I want some of the things that I feel I deserve. Even when I graduate I won't be able to get any better job than I can right now. I don't see why I should waste another year. I do enjoy studying and learning, but I can't stand the constant hassle with money. I'm here on financial aid so if I quit I probably won't ever be able to come back. I'm also tired of this place. I figure if I have to stay here one more year, I'll never make it.

Helper Responses:

1. Is there any reason why you should have to finish school at this particular university?

2. Have you looked into any alternatives to being a poverty-stricken college student in any great detail?

3. I know what you mean. It's really a rotten situation to be in.

4. You've really got a lot on your mind. Could you tell me more about where you stand in school or what the money hassle involves?

Excerpt 14

Helpee: Hi! I'm going to have a baby! Don't get shook. I'm happily married, have been for four years and we have been trying so hard for so long. It finally worked! I'm pregnant!! Since I'm sure now, I'm going to tell Jerry tonight over a candlelight dinner, his favorite dish and the whole works. I'm so happy, isn't it fantastic?

Helper Responses:

1. That's great! It *must* be a fantastic feeling to know you're going to have a baby, something you've wanted so long come true.

2. Are you sure your husband wants a baby just now?

3. It sure does sound fantastic. This is a great day for you and your husband. You'll be making a lot of new plans now, I expect.

4. Pregnancy can really be a great experience. Now you and your husband will have to make some decisions regarding how to have the baby and raise it.

Excerpt 15

Helpee: I'm having problems with my boyfriend. We've been getting pretty intimate lately, and all that is left is going all the way. I'm not sure it's what I want to do because I've always wanted to be a virgin when I got married, but it's awfully tempting. I've been brought up to believe that sex outside of marriage is wrong, but how can it be wrong when I love him so much? He doesn't understand this and is getting very impatient because I won't go all the way. I'm afraid I'll lose him if I don't, but I'm afraid I'll hate myself if I do.

Helper Responses:

1. Are you afraid of sex? Sometimes these things happen when people feel inhibited about their inner emotions.

2. It sounds like you don't know which is more important, pleasing your boyfriend and possibly yourself, or possibly losing your boyfriend for the values that even *you* are questioning.

3. That must really be a confusing situation to be in, not to know which way to go in such an important situation.

4. Why would you hate yourself for going all the way if you love him the way you say you do?

Excerpt 16

Helpee: I've been running into some people that are really messing me up. It seems like for the last few months I have been meeting nothing but Jesus freaks, the type that say "hi" and then ask if you have accepted Christ. The first few times it was interesting to rap with them, but now I'm getting tired of it, but I don't know how to politely tell them to shut up. They always end up with a rap about how stupid people are who don't accept Christ and how we were really missing out on something. At the same time, I am not sure I want to make the commitment, and I hate having it constantly shoved down my throat.

Helper Responses:

1. Sounds like you're frustrated with two problems: one, how to deal with people you don't want to be involved with and two, how to deal

with yourself, your own feelings. Let's discuss it and see if we can come up with some alternatives.

2. Why don't you tell them to be quiet and leave you alone? You don't have to let them lecture to you.

3. Do you believe in God?

4. Sounds like you're having some problems determining if you can deal with these people and with yourself as well.

TABLE II-I

KEY TO DESIGN AND RATINGS OF HELPER RESPONSES
TO HELPEE EXPRESSIONS

Helpee Expressions	Helper Responses	Facilitation	Action Orientation	Overall Rating
I	1	High	High	3.5
	2	Low	Low	1.0
	3	Low	High	2.0
	4	High	Low	3.0
II	1	Low	High	1.5
	2	High	Low	3.0
	3	Low	Low	1.0
	4	High	High	4.0
III	1	Low	Low	1.0
	2	High	High	3.5
	3	Low	High	1.5
	4	High	Low	2.5
IV	1	Low	Low	1.0
	2	Low	High	1.5
	3	High	High	3.0
	4	High	Low	2.5
V	1	High	Low	2.5
	2	Low	Low	1.0
	3	High	High	3.5
	4	Low	High	1.5
VI	1	Low	High	1.5
	2	High	High	3.5
	3	Low	Low	1.5
	4	High	Low	2.0
VII	1	High	High	3.0
	2	Low	High	1.5
	3	Low	Low	1.0
	4	High	Low	2.5
VIII	1	Low	Low	1.0
	2	Low	High	1.5
	3	High	Low	2.0
	4	High	High	3.0
IX	1	High	High	3.5
	2	High	Low	3.0
	3	Low	High	2.0
	4	Low	Low	1.0

Helpee Expressions	Helper Responses	Facilitation	Action Orientation	Overall Rating
X	1	Low	High	1.5
	2	High	High	3.0
	3	High	Low	3.0
	4	Low	Low	1.0
XI	1	High	Low	2.5
	2	Low	High	1.5
	3	High	High	3.5
	4	Low	Low	1.0
XII	1	High	High	3.5
	2	Low	Low	1.0
	3	Low	High	1.5
	4	High	Low	3.0
XIII	1	Low	Low	1.0
	2	Low	High	1.5
	3	High	Low	2.0
	4	High	High	3.0
XIV	1	High	Low	3.0
	2	Low	Low	1.0
	3	High	High	3.5
	4	Low	High	2.0
XV	1	Low	Low	1.0
	2	High	High	3.0
	3	High	Low	2.0
	4	Low	High	1.5
XVI	1	High	High	3.5
	2	Low	High	1.5
	3	Low	Low	1.0
	4	High	Low	3.0

REFERENCES

Bergin, A. E.: Some implications of psychotherapy research for therapeutic practice. *Journal of Abnormal Psychology, 21*:235-246, 1966.

Carkhuff, R. R.: *Helping and Human Relations.* New York, Holt, Rinehart and Winston, Inc., 1969, vols. I and II.

Eysenck, H. J.: The effects of psychotherapy: an evaluation. *Journal of Consulting Psychology, 16*:319-324, 1952.

McLennan, B. W. *et al.:* Training for new careers. *Community Mental Health Journal, 2*:135-141, 1966.

Pearl, A. and Riessman, F.: *New Careers for the Poor,* New York, The Free Press, 1965.

Riessman, F.: Strategies and suggestions for training nonprofessionals. *The Community Mental Health Journal, 3*(2):103-110, 1967.

Riessman, F. and Popper, H. I.: *Up from Poverty: New Career Ladders for Nonprofessionals.* New York, Harper and Row, 1968.

III

TRAINING: MAKING SURE THE HELPER IS HELPFUL

URSULA DELWORTH

ADEQUATE training coincides with appropriate selection as vital in the development of effective volunteers. Through selection we locate potentially helpful persons. Through training we maximize the chance that they will be genuinely helpful to others.

There is much information available on what centers currently are doing in terms of training, so we will start with a brief overview of training programs. Following this, a comprehensive training model will be presented.

CURRENT STATUS

Crisis centers report two main types or "times" of training—preservice (preliminary) and in-service (continuing). In many services these overlap. Some services offer no formal training.

In pre-service training, sessions range from one day or several brief sessions to courses in universities offered for credit and extending over a quarter or semester. Many of the latter are combined with in-service training. That is, volunteers begin to serve in the center during the training period. A common procedure seems to be to begin training with the policies and objectives of the center, followed by information regarding relevant dimensions of the service (drugs, sex, suicide, etc.). Often, role-playing of calls or walk-in situations is included. Community and college resources frequently are outlined.

A number of centers publish a training manual for volunteers. This can be quite comprehensive, including not only policies and procedures, but information on specific problem areas and referrals as well.

A monthly meeting seems to be the in-service training norm for crisis services, although some report holding meetings as often as once

36

a week. The group may meet as a whole, or small group meetings may be held to fit individual schedules. The content varies from opportunities to consult on difficult calls and interviews to structured training in various areas with which volunteers are expected to be familiar.

Often, new volunteers with limited (or no) pre-service experience are first given clerical or other supportive tasks to accomplish. They are allowed to work as "helpers" after they have attended a specified number of in-service sessions.

It appears that a number of centers have themselves fairly "together" regarding training. However, there is certainly no set pattern, and some evaluation and resarch is needed to determine *what kind* of training and *how much* of it is needed to prepare volunteers to operate effectively in *what type* of service. Just as we select for a specific service, we train in terms of the service to be offered.

Realizing that much still needs to be known, we would suggest a model of training which incorporates much of what currently is being done, and is additive in some areas.

A COMPREHENSIVE MODEL

What the Volunteer Needs to Know

It is probably obvious to the reader that crisis center staff members need to know some things—about people, about the environment, about current problems—in order to help others. What they need to know will vary from one center to another, depending upon services offered and clientele served. The following list is not all-inclusive, but can serve as a guide for the areas about which most staff in crisis services will need a good deal of knowledge.

1. Policies, procedures and organization of the service: objectives and limitations.

2. Drugs: currently used "hard" and "soft" drugs, alcohol, etc.; how to handle drug questions and emergencies; referrals.

3. Draft: general policies at least; referral for more detailed counseling if it is not available at the center.

4. Legal: laws that apply to crisis center services; referrals for clients to lawyers or legal aid services in the area.

5. Health: information on current health problems (VD, etc.), emergency services available, referrals for specific problems.

6. Pregnancy, birth control, and abortion: information on methods, referrals.

7. Suicide: knowledge of causes and indications; management of suicidal crisis.

8. Environment: how and where does one get help?
    a. Community: food stamps, family-child services, all medical-legal services, public school services and programs, child care services, religious groups, etc.
    b. Campus: registration, academic problems, financial aid, student organizations, all medical-legal services, etc.

9. Resources: Volunteers can't know everything, but they need to know key persons in the community/campus who can answer questions and help make specific referrals.

10. Potential clients or helpees of the service: What kinds of problems may they present? What needs to be known about their life styles and functioning?

11. Self-knowledge: Who am I? What are my own hang-ups and biases which may get in the way of offering effective service?

How Can the Volunteer Learn These Things?

Areas one through nine above especially lend themselves to a didactic approach, that is, to some sort of presentation by a knowledgable person. Here it is important that the "expert" not only know what he is talking about, but be able to communicate effectively with his audience. A dull lecture is about the worst way to try to get a point across!

Reading often proves to be a viable avenue of gaining information. The condensed versions of problem areas found in some training manuals can be especially helpful. Selecting and condensing useful material (with permission, of course) seems to be an economical and effective way to train volunteers in any number of vital subject areas. Many manuals contain at least an information section on drugs and suicide.

If reading is the method utilized to cover certain areas, then discussion of content and implication for the crisis service should follow. (This is best done in small groups, to give each person a chance, and the responsibility, to contribute his ideas.)

Visits to referral agencies and/or meetings with agency staff will help volunteers feel more comfortable in referring persons to those services. If there are many such agencies, perhaps several trainees could visit each and report on their impressions to the group.

A good knowledge of relevant fields will stand the volunteer in good stead in all situations. Indeed, in some services he will many times be called upon for little else than his informational expertise.

But learning how to handle crisis situations goes far beyond learning their causation or the resources available to the person. The volunteer needs to assimilate this knowledge and use it in a manner which allows him to "tune in" to the person in crisis, and to work with him toward resolution of the problem.

Here we come to the problem of how to develop the effective helper, the person who can really "make a difference." The technique of interviewing serves as something of a bridge between cognitive and effective (feeling) learning. The volunteer has to know what to ask, and how to ask it, either on the phone or in a walk-in situation. Most centers train heavily around the interview, starting with a general approach to help the client feel some confidence in the service. Specific questions to ask and topics to cover in various problem areas are then covered. There are a number of approaches which can be used to help the volunteer integrate and begin to utilize the information he has gained.

Role-playing is a basic method to practice the interview model. This gives the volunteer an opportunity to act in as helpful a manner as he can, receive feedback on how he is coming across, and then modify his approach accordingly. (Some centers attempt to accomplish this by putting new volunteers right into the service situation, and then critiquing their performance with them. This has obvious "reality" advantages, but raises questions concerning the client's right to the best possible help from a fully trained staff member.) One of the values in role-playing is the chance for the trainee to take the "helpee" role, and respond to the kind of help his fellow trainees give him.

Reading can help in learning to be an effective helper as well as in specific content fields. "Telephone Therapy: Some Common Errors and Fallacies," by Charles W. Lamb (1970), is one good article in this area.

Another approach incorporates personal growth experiences as a tool. T-groups or encounter groups are used here to give the volunteer an opportunity to grow as an individual and to learn to communicate more effectively with others. This can be useful, provided the trainee is helped to transfer this added insight into how he functions as a crisis center volunteer.

A number of approaches to this difficult problem are currently in use by crisis services. Two of these, both from university centers, are presented briefly. Two more general approaches which can be utilized for crisis training are presented as well.

Suicidology Model

Volunteers at the University of Northern Colorado take the three credit-hour class "Suicidology: Crisis Intervention," which includes a lecture session, a small group seminar session weekly and a six-hour shift of the phones about twice every three weeks. The volunteers are trained to handle calls from persons who are suicidal. The heart of the training centers around the five steps outlined in the *Training Manual for Telephone Evaluation and Emergency Management of Suicidal Persons* (see Chapter X). These steps are: (a) establishing a relationship, maintaining contact, and obtaining information, (b) identification and clarification of the focal problem(s), (c) evaluation of the suicidal potential, (d) assessment of the strength and resources, and (e) formulation of a therapy plan and mobilization of patient's and others' resources.

The first two steps are readily adaptable to all other kinds of problems which might be phoned in. Thus, this portion of the suicidology model of training can be applied to all other kinds of problems. Role-playing among trainees is heavily emphasized to teach the first two steps. Steps (d) and (e) can also apply to a variety of other kinds of calls and a large amount of class time is spent in presenting various persons from many of the resource agencies in the Greeley area. These may include representatives of the police, county mental health clinic, physicians, birth control information center, draft information center, drug information and referral center, veterans' counselor, ministers, lawyers.

A good deal of time is spent talking about suicide because it is the most frightening kind of call with which a volunteer could be presented. Once these fears are allayed through training, the volunteer hopefully becomes less fearful of phone duty and becomes more effective in all his duties.

The most recent trend in training at the center is to get away from talking about suicide as much as was previously done. The trainers are stressing the wide applicability of the five steps to other kinds of problems.

UNC served as a participant last year in a pilot curriculum prepared by the Center for the Study of Suicide Prevention at the National Institute of Mental Health. NIMH provided a number of training aids and references. Information regarding the pilot curriculum and materials are available through

Dr. H. L. P. Resnik, Chief
Center for the Studies of Suicide Prevention
National Institute of Mental Health
Chevy Chase, Md. 20015

Further information on the UNC program is available through

Dr. David Smart
Counseling Center
University of Northern Colorado
Greeley, Colorado 80631

Core Dimensions Model

RoadHouse, crisis/information calling service at Colorado State University, offers a two-unit special studies course in psychology to students who have been selected as prospective volunteers. The training process consists of the following phases:

PHASE I, CONTENT AREAS. This is training in the informational areas with which a volunteer needs to be familiar. The areas are covered previously in this chapter. Since RoadHouse services both university and community, resources in both areas are covered. This training is given mostly through talks by informed persons.

PHASE II, CORE DIMENSIONS. The dimensions of the helping relationship, as articulated by Robert Carkhuff (1969) are presented. These include empathy, genuineness, and confrontation. Following this overview in the large group of 30 to 40 persons, students are divided into subgroups of six to eight students. These groups are led by student trainers. Here each specific dimension is presented, discussed and practiced.

At first the training is concentrated on helping the prospective volunteer give good initial responses. As students become more familiar with the dimension in question, more extended practice is given. That is, a longer portion of the interview is role-played.

PHASE III, INTEGRATION. Students, again in their small groups, are asked to role-play typical interview situations. Here they are expected to be able to use both the information learned in Phase I, what to say, and the helping dimensions, how to say it. The closing part of this phase involves mock phone calls which each student trainer first presents to the persons in his group and which he then evaluates with them.

Most volunteers are scheduled on the phones at the end of training. Some few are given extended training in one or another area. Once in a while, a volunteer needs help in sorting out his own personal concerns which are interfering with his ability to be helpful to others. Such persons are referred to an appropriate agency for counseling.

RoadHouse has recently begun to administer the Carkhuff Communication Index and the Crisis Center Communication Index as pre-training and post-training measures. (These indexes consist of helpee excerpts and an initial response from the volunteer. See chapter on *selection* for a more complete account.) The main purpose here is evaluation of training, but it also seems that dealing with typical problem situations prior to training increases the student's sensitivity to areas in which he has difficulty giving responses. He can then especially work on these areas during training.

Further information can be obtained from:

Janet Taub
RoadHouse
Colorado State University
Fort Collins, Colorado 80521

Creative Listening

This approach has been developed by the Creative Listeners Guild. A staff member, Myldred E. Jones, is a pioneer in the crisis center/ hotline movement and is utilizing this technique with crisis services.

The CLG group states the following regarding their program.

Our training objective is to enable each participant, through the creative listening process, to discover and use those resources within himself that have not as yet been touched, freeing him to become a more responsive and self-fulfilling human being in his work, in his home and in his community.

Specifically, each participant will:

. . . discover that he is allowing his preconceptions and built-in prejudices to interfere with his response to others, that he neither fully understands, nor is fully understood.

. . . examine his motives and feelings about relationships and issues in his personal and professional life, and how these prompt judgmental responses.

. . . experience listening creatively.

. . . evaluate his gain. (Creative Listeners Guild, 1971)

Specific information on this approach can be obtained by writing to

Myldred E. Jones
Creative Listeners Guild
1506 South Bay Front
Balboa Island, California 92662

Basic Helping Skills Program

This model for training paraprofessionals (which can include crisis center volunteers) has been developed by Steven J. Danish. The Basic Helping Skills Program is designed to assist paraprofessional trainees in learning how to become more effective helpers. This program focuses upon three basic components of helping: (a) self-understanding, (b) knowledge of some of the helping strategies or techniques, and (c) practice and experience in applying these strategies.

The procedure used to teach most of the skills is to (a) define the skill or ability to be learned, (b) discuss the need for learning this skill, (c) give examples of the skill, (d) specify the level of achievement necessary so both student and instructor are confident that the student has achieved, (e) practice the skill, including homework and (f) become acquainted with the next skill to be learned.

There are ten separate sections of the Basic Helping Skills Program. Further information on the entire course can be obtained from

Dr. Steven J. Danish
Counseling and Testing Center
Southern Illinois University
Carbondale, Illinois 62901

Who Should Train?

As discussed in the chapter on selection, only those persons should serve as trainers who are more skilled or knowledgeable in the area to be taught than are the trainees. This seems self-evident, but is a far from universally followed rule. Robert Carkhuff emphasizes the importance of this rule when he states, "If the trainer is functioning at high levels of the dimensions on which the trainee is being trained, the probability of the success of training with any trainee population is high." (Carkhuff, 1971, p. 185).

Carkhuff and others also stress the necessity for the trainer to be a good model for the persons whom he trains. Thus, in a crisis service situation, the trainer should exhibit the helpful attitudes and skills with the trainees which he later expects them to use as volunteers.

It seems especially important to have persons who can serve as good models as trainers in the experiential phase of training, that is, the phase in which the trainees are learning to use the skills and information which they have been previously taught. Persons presenting information in the specific problem areas primarily need valid and thorough knowledge in the area and ability to get the information across to others. It is even better if, in addition, they can serve as models of helping persons in their relationship with trainees. Trainers also need the ability to *teach,* to impart knowledge and skills to others. They may be excellent as volunteers and/or professionals, but the training function requires that they can actively communicate their knowledge to the trainees as well.

With these criteria in mind, we can look for our trainers in a variety of places. Members of the governing or advisory boards of the center may be able to help. Professionals from any number of community agencies may be well-informed about specific topics and willing to present them to the training group.

A core group of trainers who will help the trainees to integrate information and practices by whatever approach used, probably should be formed. This group then becomes responsible for the experiential portion of the training. It can certainly include professionals. A professional probably would, in fact, conduct the initial training for the core group itself. However, it makes sense to have some, if not all, of the core members be members of the nonprofessional crisis center staff. Modeling of helpful approaches by such persons may be more believable and real to the trainees. Also, this is a good utilization of trained staff—allowing them part of the training role. In some centers, nonprofessional staff conduct all of the training, with only minor consultation with professionals. This seems to be a "mature model," one which a center can utilize after it has been operating long enough to have various persons with high skill levels as part of the staff.

REFERENCES

Carkhuff, R. R.: *Helping and Human Relations.* New York, Holt, Rinehart and Winston, Inc., 1969, vols. I and II.

Carkhuff, R. R.: Principles of social action in training for new careers in human services. *Journal of Counseling Psychology, 18*(2):147-151, 1971.

Carkhuff, R. R.: *The Development of Human Resources.* New York, Holt, Rinehart and Winston, Inc., 1971.

Lamb, C. W.: Telephone therapy: some common errors and fallacies. *Voices, 5*(4):42-46, 1969-1970.

IV

FINANCING TIPS FOR CRISIS CENTERS
AND HOTLINES

Edward H. Rudow and Bernie Gebhardt

THEORETICALLY, there should be no difficulty in obtaining finances for the maintenance of a crisis center or hotline within an average sized community. With the growing recognition by the general citizenry of the increasing problems of drug abuse, social alienation and family breakdown among people, it would seem that there should be a parallel growth in the willingness of the community to help solve these problems.

But time after time in countless communities across the nation, crisis centers and calling lines have been forced to discontinue their oftentimes highly commendable operations due to inadequate finances. Therefore, the following will hopefully offer a few helpful observations, hints and reminders for those of you involved with the financial aspects of starting and maintaining such centers or hotlines.

The first thing you should be aware of in trying to secure fundings for your project is that nobody is going to finance an ill-planned, partially thought out, disorganized pipe dream. Your project must be totally clear in your own mind. You should have as many facts and figures, specific examples and witnesses as you can to show why your project is needed. You must be able, in writing, to clearly articulate the problem which your service is meant to help resolve; show its various roots; demonstrate its predictable future; explain the advantages and disadvantages of your approach to the problem. Nobody is going to believe you, and rightfully so, if you try to convince them that you have the final answer or that you have all the answers to the problem. Be honest with yourself and with others from the very beginning about the goals and methods of your project. This is extremely important, so that your financial backers will not drop out after a short while because you did not solve all of the community's problems overnight. Most importantly, however, you must remain honest from the beginning about your capabilities and expectations so that you yourself will not become disenchanted when the difficulties mount up.

If your proposed service has true merit, however, and you have been able to show a need for it within your community, financial backers can eventually be found. Remember, no matter how or by what means you raise funds, the most important thing to consider is that you must have a product to sell. You must be able to show in a simple and straightforward fashion how you are going to operate, when you are going to operate, what your objectives are, and again, that there is a definite need for your service. If there is not a need for your services, it might be better to get a job as a shoe salesman than to try to create the need.

Now to some of the details: for what, specifically, will you need finances? It becomes evident soon after beginning a service, that it takes more than warm bodies to keep the center in operation. Material costs arise from every direction from the very beginning. Before the doors open, there must be a door to open—you have to have a facility. You can buy one, rent one, or find one that is free, whichever is easiest. Churches, schools, business clubs, fraternal lodges, are all good places to check when seeking a facility. Once you have a place, you need furnishings—desks, chairs, tables, etc. You can rough most of it, with pillows and boxes and borrowed chairs and tables. There are a great many odds and ends that do not cost money and that, with a little imagination, can look fine.

Next, office equipment must be considered. A typewriter might seem an extravagant expense, but if you have ever had to decipher someone else's handwriting, or if you want to write a business letter, you soon discover the necessity for one. Pens, pencils, paper, stationery, envelopes, stamps and erasers are small but necessary items. If you are going to keep records, you are going to need some type of filing system and a file cabinet, preferably one with a lock, for confidential matters. You will find that a duplicating machine will be most helpful for keeping your volunteers posted and sending out community notices and articles. A duplicating machine or access to one is almost a must. You might also want to consider a bulletin board for posting messages and announcements.

Whether you are operating strictly a phone service or a walk-in center, you are going to need telephone equipment, a small switchboard, at least. Expect to pay considerably more than you do for the service charge on your home phone. Some centers report that they have received contributions from their local phone companies equivalent to the costs of their phone expense; this is the exception rather than the rule. One thing you can check into is the charity rate which is given to churches. This amounts to a percentage reduction on the service charge on your main phone, and though it is not a large amount, it helps.

Now that you have an office, equipment, supplies and furnishings, and your staff, you are almost ready to begin, but not quite yet. Your volunteers have to be trained and trained correctly. Training materials, including books, films, and speakers, cost money. Some of the materials can be obtained free or at a nominal cost from the government or some public agency, but there are still ones you will have to buy. In addition, after your people are trained they will still need new and up-dated reference material, books and speakers. These people are the core of your organization. Treat them well; keep them informed.

It should also be realized that while most centers are manned by volunteers, someone is needed to supervise the total operation. This individual may have to spend a considerable amount of time keeping up with his work. In many cases it can amount to more than a full-time job. This of course raises the question of compensation for the director. Directors receive various amounts of salary depending on their qualifications, workload and scope of operation of the project. In addition, it is often necessary to hire a full-time secretary to insure continuity of office operations.

Finally, when you have a place with phones, materials and trained people, you are ready to meet the public. Now people must learn about you and your intended services. Your publicity can take many forms: handouts, posters, newspaper ads, radio spots, and word of mouth; however, all but the last cost money. The best means of publicity are your own personal contacts with the local kids.

All of the above are essential items and materials necessary for the operation of a center. Some other things which come in handy are a coffee pot, a pan for boiling water, coffee, tea, cocoa, sugar, dry cream, things to help you through the early morning hours. You might also want to consider subscriptions to the local newspaper and possibly a radio.

If after having read the above you are still determined to open a center, we recommend that your organization incorporate as a non-profit corporation. Also file with the Internal Revenue Service as a tax-exempt organization. These two acts are separate; becoming a nonprofit corporation does not automatically entitle you to tax exemptions. You can file for the first through your state and the second through the federal government. This is best handled by an attorney. There are several advantages of being a nonprofit corporation with tax-exempt status: (a) you do not have to pay sales tax on merchandise for the center's operation; (b) any contributions made to your organization are tax deductible items for the contributors; (c) any money received is not taxable, and (d) you can more easily apply for grant money. If you are going to operate on a college campus as a recognized student organization, incorporation may not be necessary. Check with your school administration to see if you are covered by the school's own status.

As a corporation, you are going to need a board of directors. The matter of selecting the board should not be taken lightly. There are two basic considerations. The first is that the board members can be of some considerable assistance, as outside interested individuals, in helping your organization to thrive both professionally and financially. Secondly, they can also help to cut costs in some areas. A way to save lawyer fees, for instance, is to place an interested attorney on your board. He can help you not only with the incorporation papers, but with the many numerous legal questions and problems which will arise. Lawyers are constantly being approached for voluntary legal service, so they are expecting you; tell the truth about why you want them.

Another good board appointment along this line would be an individual who has experience in writing grant proposals. There are numerous agencies which have money available for operations such as a crisis center, but even with the best program in the world, you can not tap these resources unless you have someone, a grantsman, who can communicate with the agencies. Often, the grantsman serves as an interpreter, so that all parties involved understand the procedures. It would be beneficial, then, if the interpreter were on your side.

Your board should include one or two businessmen from the community. These people not only lend respectability to your organization, but are also familiar with sources of revenue within the community. They might also sponsor advertising for your project on the local radio stations or in the paper. It would be easiest, of course, if you could get the local newspaper publisher on your board.

Professionals who could do some of your voluteer training would also make good board members. They can save you the cost of having to hire someone to assist in your training program.

To round out your board, you should try to acquire someone who is familiar and active with other charitable organizations. His experience could save you from making many mistakes which other organizations have made.

Remember that the lawyer, the doctor, the grantsman and the businessman, not to mention the publisher, have been approached before. If you want their help, your presentation must be a convincing one. It is always preferable that people gladly give their help and time because they feel that they are needed for what they are and what they can do, rather than for whom they know and what they have done.

If you do not incorporate because you are a campus student organization, you will not need a board of directors as such, but an advisory board should be formed in its stead. If applicable, the advisory board should have a composition representative of the university, similar to the cross-community representation on the board of directors.

Let us now turn to some ways to obtain working capital. The first consideration is the possibility of obtaining a grant from somebody. Grants can be obtained from a number of agencies: federal, state, local and private. Two excellent books which list sources of grants are *The Foundation Directory* (1967) and *The Annual Register of Grant Support* (1971). Grants may be awarded for any number of reasons: training, community health development, crime prevention, drug treatment and rehabilitation and research, just to mention a few. Helpful pointers for prospective grant recipients are: (a) find the important issues at the present time, for example, law enforcement and drug treatment and prevention are currently hot topics and, (b) demonstrate to the granting agency that your operation is directly involved with the most prevalent issues of the day.

You should be aware that it is possible to receive grants from more than one agency. For example, if you are operating a crisis center which caters to a variety of different problems, you may be able to receive partial support from the National Institute of Mental Health under their community mental health centers staffing section and at the same time receive additional support from one of the agencies handling money made available from the Omnibus Crime Control and Safe Streets acts.

Too often people seeking grant support think only of large federal agencies (e.g. the Department of Health, Education and Welfare, and the National Science Foundation). They tend to forget that there are similar state agencies which may have funds available. Similarly, many people are well acquainted with some of the large, private foundations, such as the Rockefeller Foundation and the Ford Foundation, but many people are not aware that there are many small, local foundations, some confined within the community itself. In one relatively small town, population approximately 40,000, the local crisis center was surprised to learn that there were two such foundations.

The problem with obtaining grants is that they are often difficult to get, and are a long time coming when they are awarded. As mentioned previously, it takes an individual experienced with grantsmanship to do an effective job in making the contact. And if you do receive a grant, there are usually some strings attached as to how, where and when you may use the funds. This might mean giving up some autonomy, but if you have told the truth about what your really intend to do, the rewards usually outweigh the costs.

Another more immediate method of raising funds is similar to getting a grant, but on a smaller scale and not quite as formal. If you believe that your crisis center is needed, you may be able to convince other related agencies that your service could be a worthy addition to their own. Since you are going to have to make a list of the helping agencies for referral purposes, you can use this same list for potential sources of funds. Included in this list should be such agencies as the local mental health center, the social welfare department, the hospital, the medical society, local law enforcement agencies, etc. You will find that some of these agencies will claim that they do not have enough funds for their own operations. While this may be true, you do not need to accept it as final fact. Most agencies have some type of contingency fund from which they can draw. Even if they can give you relatively little, it can serve as a beginning.

Churches can also be a good source for funds and/or facilities. They often have space which is vacant most of the week which you may be able to use as a location for your operation; this can save a considerable amount in rent and utilities. If you approach them correctly, you can also obtain some money from their general treasury. One good technique is to demonstrate how beneficial your program is in helping youth and that surely they could allocate a portion of their youth fund toward your operation. If you can get nothing else, at least ask for their endorsement. It is good public relations and can eliminate a lot of criticism, while aiding in raising funds from private citizens.

Other good sources of revenue are your local service clubs, fraternal organizations, and business associations. These organizations which do not have large treasuries from which to draw may wish to help in some sort of service capacity. In one town the less affluent organizations joined together in an attempt to raise money for the operation of a drug crisis and information center. These same clubs may also provide volunteers to work either in direct operation of the center or as aides in handling administrative details (e.g. addressing envelopes, making phone calls, cleaning and painting).

Some groups involved with the operation of running a crisis center have developed a novel way of getting contributions from private citizens. Instead of asking for contributions, they ask people to become members of an organization which sponsors their efforts. These people, in order to join the organization, pay an initiation fee and annual dues in return they are given restricted voting privileges in selecting a board of directors for the operation. How many and what types of privileges these people are afforded depends on the amount of autonomy you are willing to relinquish.

There are numerous projects which take relatively little time, but can bring in additional revenue. Many organizations as part of their fund-raising have gone out and collected aluminum cans and sold them as part of the recycling, ecology movement. You might want to spend one day every month or so doing this and in-between time make available locations around town where people can deposit cans.

One group spent an afternoon going door-to-door, but insted of asking for money they solicited deposit-type soda pop and milk bottles. People are generally responsive to this because they are not only helping, but getting a service performed for them since nobody likes to take bottles back.

Another project which can be undertaken is to sell car bumper stickers or window decals. The scale of these items helps not only to raise funds but to serve as good publicity for the center since they begin appearing all over the town.

One college center was given a waterbed by a local merchant. They in turn sold raffle tickets for the waterbed and were able to raise some needed monies. A word of caution here concerning raffles: different states and cities have varying laws pertaining to the sale, distribution and accounting of raffle tickets, so be sure to check with a lawyer before undertaking a project like this.

There is an old traditional "carwash" when your volunteers get together and offer to wash peoples' cars at a minimal cost. This area has been heavily cut into by the new automated car washes, but one group has found a way around this. They have made a deal with one of the local car washes. They will send people to his establishment if they get 10 percent cut of the cost of the wash from anyone who mentions they were sent by the center. You might try this with other merchants. It should work well in any highly competitive market area or with new businessmen who are trying to become known.

One group of people obtained the cooperation of a local radio station and ran a 53-hour marathon. This is a good way to make money. The purpose of the marathon was to raise funds for the crisis center and also to inform the local community about the project and the operation. While they were on the air they solicited merchandise from the local merchants to be auctioned over the radio. Naturally the merchandise was free and any price paid for it was clear profit. Additional benefit of the marathon was that people became familiar with the project and it took less persuasion in future fund-raising campaigns to get them to contribute.

Those centers which operate on a college or university campus have some additional sources of revenue. They may, for example, receive recognition as a bona fide student organization and thereby be allowed to receive allocations from the student government. There are a number of other ways of tapping into the university treasury. For example, they can approach the administration and ask to receive money directly from the president's or vice-president's office for student relations, or they may approach one of the dean's offices or the student personnel administrators. One other source that campus groups may turn to are the alumni associations. You can approach either the office directly or solicit contributions from individual graduates. If you represent a campus group, do not be discouraged if you are told that your fund requests have been refused the first time. Remember, there is always money to be had through an administrative office. Just keep trying.

In conclusion, the financing of any worthwhile project is always its least glamorous side. To make financing the most important aspect of the project would be a tremendous mistake, for the emphasis must always remain on providing assistance for those who seek it. The community does have a feeling for itself, and for what is truly a service to itself. It is by performing your service humbly and well that you can be assured of adequate financial support for your endeavors. In simple words, help and you will be helped. Is this not the concept upon which the crisis centers are based?

REFERENCES

Lewis, M. O. (Ed.) : *The Foundation Directory*. New York, Russell Sage Foundation, 1967.

Renetzky, A. (Ed.) : *Annual Register of Grant Support*. Orange, New Jersey, Academic Media, 1971.

V

LEGAL CONSIDERATIONS IN CRISIS CENTER OPERATIONS

PENFIELD TATE AND CHARLOTTE GREENFIELD

WHEN individuals prepare to establish a crisis center their legal rights and responsibilities must not be overlooked. Therefore, one of the first efforts should be aimed toward establishing liaison with an attorney in the immediate area, one who will be aware of the applicability of the various laws, both statutory and judicial, to the operation of a crisis center. If the crisis center is to be operated under the wing of a college or university, church, or public agency, the legal staff of that parent organization must be made a part of the early planning, since it will most probably be the parent organization which is held responsible for the activities of the center. Private attorneys can be contacted through the local bar association, both to find an attorney for the center and to draw up a referral list for clients needing legal advice.

It would be wise at the outset to indicate that the laws to which crisis centers will be held accountable will vary from state to state; thus legal advice must be sought from someone versed in the law of the state involved. There are, however, some generalities in the law which will prevail throughout the country. In this chapter we will address ourselves to some of these.

CONFIDENTIAL INFORMATION

When one is dealing with an individual seeking counsel, and information of a personal nature is passed from one to another, questions of privacy and confidentiality arise. Generally speaking, all staff members, professional and nonprofessional personnel alike, have a duty to their clients to disclose personal and private information only in a bona fide effort to help that client, and then only to the extent necessary. Of course, this covers the nonprofessional staff member giving information to a therapist, doctor or lawyer for counseling purposes. The ethical canons of the medical profession and the legal profession are examples of the standards set up to protect the relationships that can only function effectively in an atmosphere of trust. Nonprofessionals on the staff are bound only by the crisis center rules concerning confidential information and their own personal code of conduct. Because of this it is important that any operating procedures firmly state the requirement for strict confidentiality by nonprofessional personnel regarding any information reaching him through his crisis center participation. If these standards are violated to the detriment of a client, the client may always initiate a suit in libel or for invasion of privacy against the individual and the center. The center is in a much better legal position when it is clear that the violation was made in conflict with its existing operating procedures.

However, there are potential situations which may exert pressure upon staff members to involuntarily divulge confidential information: inquiries from public officials—police, welfare department, probation or parole officers. In keeping with the trust placed in the crisis center staff by their clients, each center must develop guidelines for dealing with these situations. So long as the request for information is informal, that is by telephone or letter, all public officials may (legally) be refused access to records or to information known to a staff member, if that is the decision of the center or the staff member.

Public agencies or officials have another option at their disposal. They may receive a subpoena from a court of competent jurisdiction to require that they be given the information they want and/or they may require that a crisis center employee appear as a witness in an action. Once the public agency or official obtains a subpoena, or the crisis center staff member is called as a witness in a formal court proceeding, the legal right to refuse to divulge confidential information without the consent of the client depends upon the state statutes and decisions regulating what information may be kept confidential in a court setting. These statutes set up what is known as a "privilege" to refuse to answer questions which impinge on the confidential relationship that the witness has had with a client. By and large this privilege is limited to members of certain defined professions: medical doctors, psychiatrists, clergymen, or lawyers. The privilege can only be invoked by the client. If he desires to waive the privilege, the professional has no choice but to testify. Others, including nonprofessional staff members in a crisis center as well as social workers, have no legal protection. Therefore all questions pertinent to the matter being determined in court must be answered by these persons even though private information is thereby divulged. Furthermore, even professionals protected in this manner under statutes must have an understanding of what types of information are covered—the privilege is a limited one. Courts in every state have strictly construed the statutory privileges that do exist—largely for the reason that they impede the court's "search for truth." Once again, however, these applications of the statute are different in every state, so that consultation with your local attorney is in order.*

Where counseling by a member of one of these professions is not called for, some measure of privacy can be provided by a technique employed by at least one operating crisis center. Each client is offered the opportunity to be known by a fictitious name. The practice often has the beneficial effect of easing communication between a crisis center staff person and a client, for the very reason that the client understands that greater confidentiality results. Another technique is the use of first names only by either the client or the staff member or both. Both techniques tend to decrease the ability of either party to identify the other and thereby directly decrease the possibility of either being required to testify.

Other directors of crisis centers have determined that the risk of being forced in court to divulge information is so small, that the trusting relationship is not impinged by this possibility, and no precautions such as the use of fictitious names are taken.

ILLEGAL ACTIVITIES

It is perhaps obvious, but no harm is done by pointing out that every crisis center must insure that nothing illegal is done on the premises. Some proportion of the persons needing assistance will in one way or other be involved with illegal drugs, abortions not sanctioned under the law, or by seeking legal help after being arrested for criminal law violations. The crisis center staff, to insure the continuance of the program, if not for any other reason, must not sanction any criminal activity, particularly in the center building itself.

---

*See 71 *Yale Law Journal* 1226 (1962).

INSURANCE

A crisis center, like every business or agency open to the public, should make adequate provision to protect itself and its patrons by obtaining insurance against the risks of personal injury on the premises, fire and theft. A check should be made with the legal representative of the university or public agency that sponsors the crisis center, if any, to ascertain if adequate coverage is provided by general insurance policies to cover the center's operation. Independent centers must assess their own needs, again with the aid of an attorney.

One question often posed is whether an independent crisis center should incorporate under the state laws to protect individual staff members from individual liability. Incorporation does not, in any legal sense, relieve a staff member whose advice or actions cause injury. An injured party can sue the individual or the individual and the corporation.

The practical advantage to an injured plaintiff, of having an incorporated entity to sue as an alternate to suing the individual agent or employee or in addition to suing the individual, is that the corporation is apt to have a deeper pocket. That is the corporation will probably have more money with which to pay damages. Ninety percent of damage claims are settled out of court by negotiation—namely, between representatives of an injured person and the center's insurance company. Since both incorporated and unincorporated centers may obtain insurance, the advantage of one course or the other is not clear.

GIVING ADVICE

Another area in which the law may be stated generally is the responsibility of a crisis center for advice given by a staff member. The two hypothetical situations which follow will help to explain the possible legal consequences for a crisis center.

Suppose a young woman calls the crisis center and asks for information pertaining to an abortion. Abortions are illegal in that state except for certain specified reasons which do not apply to the facts as she relates them. Suppose further that the crisis center has a list of doctors who will perform abortions, and the young woman is given one or more names. The abortion is performed, and the young woman has subsequent medical problems and she sues the crisis center along with the doctor. Chances are better than average that a suit against the crisis center would result in a monetary award to the woman. The point of this hypothetical situation is simply that when information is provided, and injury results, the crisis center can be held responsible for the injury.

To follow this situation out to the extreme the same facts may give rise in some states to criminal responsibility. The principle is this: one who supplies another with the wherewithall to commit a crime also commits a crime himself. The crisis center has not only committed a wrong against the woman, but by statute has also committed a wrong against the state, i.e. a crime.

In the second case, suppose a woman contacts the crisis center having decided to get an abortion. It appears that she does not meet the requirements of the state abortion statute, and she is seeking information on the feasibility of obtaining a legal abortion in some other state with a more liberal abortion statute. At the outset a crisis center should have a set policy on the giving out of this type of information— the policy having been set after consulting an attorney. In parallel circumstances, for instance, a few attorneys have been reprimanded and even disbarred for advising a client to change legal residency in order to take advantage of a more liberal divorce law of another state. The result of either course of action is to undermine the effect in the home state of strict laws regulating either abortion or marriage. For that reason, advice of this nature may not always be viewed as impartial imparting of factual information.

Both hypothetical situations illustrate the difference between providing a caller with information by which he or she can implement a decision already made. In the former the possibility of liability by the crisis center is extremely small. In the latter the possibility is greatly increased.

In general, therefore, crisis center staff members would be well advised to follow this rule: Give no advice unless you are qualified to give it. Thus, only doctors or nurses should give medical advice and only lawyers can give legal advice, However, in this connection it will be helpful to many clients to have a set of your own statutes in the office. Quoting existing law, without interpretation, is not giving advice. Some crisis centers have on the premises the Red Cross first aid manuals, and use them in the same manner, that is, merely quoting what the manual says on a certain subject.

In this connection, when the client requesting assistance or advice is a minor, the best legal advice to a crisis center is—*hands off*. For all intents and purposes a minor in most states is an individual under eighteen years of age, in others it is the traditional age of twenty-one. Some particular statutes, for example abortion statutes, may specify some other age of consent. Your local attorney and your state statutes should alert you to these situations. For example the statutes of Washington specify that no person under eighteen years of age may be treated by a doctor or dentist without written parental consent, and the same requirement applies to any visit to a counselor (including psychiatric or legal) beyond the first diagnostic visit. Exceptions are made for the persons over sixteen years old seeking pregnancy tests or birth control supplies, and for persons over fourteen years old seeking diagnosis and treatment of venereal disease.* Where consulting the parents is in order, keep in mind that the original contact was made with the minor—and he or she is your client. Contact parents only with your client's consent.

Some minors coming to the attention of the crisis center will be runaways. A policy of helping such a person only on the condition that parents are contacted is often in practice. This makes sense in the light of the restrictions listed above, and is applicable even to such limited help as providing a place to "crash" for a day or so. In instances of a minor's unwillingness to call home, the parents must not necessarily be told of the minors whereabouts, but they should be told that the minor is in good health and safe.

A few minors, in certain circumstances, may be "emancipated," or responsible for themselves as if they had reached majority age. Most states treat minors who are either married or in the armed forces as emancipated. Before a staff member proceeds to treat an underage client as emancipated, the particular facts should be related to the center's attorney so that he can make the legal determination first.

This chapter has outlined the legal responsibilities of operating a crisis center and appears to be urging caution at every turn. However, we would like to conclude with an optimistic note. The scope of permissible activities by crisis center members seems quite restricted; however, that scope, and the helpful impact on your clients, can be broadened by the inclusion of professionals in the crisis center staff. If

---

*Revised Code of Washington 70.24.110 (venereal disease); 71.24.020 (Section 8) (treatment for addiction).

we were to recommend any one course of action, it would be to provide professional assistance, medical, legal or psychiatric.

In order to become familiar with the legal aspects of operating a crisis center, one should acquaint himself with state statutes regarding this type of operation. Such information would be available at a law school library, in your nearest county library, state or federal courthouse, and at the office of your attorney. Laws with which you should be particularly concerned are those dealing with the areas of (a) abortion, (b) drug possession and sale, (c) venereal disease prevention and diagnosis, and (d) doctor/patient and attorney/client privileges. Find a general discussion of privilege in 71 *Yale Law Journal* 1226 (1962).

VI

THE NITTY-GRITTY OF
CENTER OPERATIONS

JANET TAUB

T HERE are many ways to conduct the actual operations of a
center. Some are practical for all centers, while others are
tailored to specific areas. Each center has its own goals and limitations
and is unique in the problems it will face. Therefore not *all* policies or
ideas will fit *all* centers. Particularly if you are just beginning and
organizing a center, you must realize that the ideas presented here,
diverse as they may be, can have variations in themselves. They may
be changed to fit a center's specific needs.

GOVERNING STRUCTURE

A variety of methods are available for governing a center. One
that many centers use is an individual directorship. This is how many
centers were started. Someone decided to open a center, and because
he originally organized everything and set operations in motion, he
became the overall director.

An advantage of this is that when problems arise or new ideas
emerge, one knows who should be consulted about them. The director,
knowing about the center's operations, can then make a decision. If
any group wants information on the center, only the director need be
notified. If legal problems arise, the director is responsible for them,
and so on.

This structure has its obvious drawbacks as well as advantages.
Depending upon how extensive operations are, the job of being the
director is almost always a full-time job. The director is responsible
for everything that happens at the center. He or she is responsible for
training volunteers, ascertaining that information is not false or out-
dated, keeping in contact with referral agencies, and such activities.
Of course, many of these jobs may be handled by someone other than

the director, but basically they all fall under his direction. If the director is a student, a working person, or a housewife, the time the center will demand may take up equally as much and *more* time than the individual's other responsibilities.

Some centers are run by several persons who are a regular part of the organization. Responsibilities are divided, giving each person fewer obligations than those of the full-time director.

The responsibilities may be divided among any number of persons. However, a small group is advisable, to avoid having too many loose ends. Some centers have divided the directorship into three areas: finance, office operations-scheduling, and publicity and public relations work. Meetings are arranged weekly so that problems, ideas, or changes may be discussed. Despite their major areas of work, these people can be freely approached by anyone in the organization who wishes to discuss any area of the operations. The weekly meeting that these three directors have may or may not be open to the rest of the organization, according to the wishes of directors. There may be a problem the directors want to solve before the general populace becomes involved, but on the other hand, a volunteer may have an idea or problem he wants to discuss with the director. This type of communication should be encouraged.

A problem which is inherent in this system is that unless these three, or however many members, are able to work well together, communication is strained and poor. The organization then suffers. Also, unless each person does his own job, someone else must take up the responsibilities. None of the three areas listed can go unattended. Honest communication is a must!

Other centers operate under a board of directors from the community. This board may be made up of members of the community— housewife to bank president. If a university is involved, the board may be made up of university personnel, or university and community members. Under this system, the board has the overall responsibility and decides the policies of the center. Its members may be responsible for different areas, eg. finance, or it may appoint someone in the organization to handle these tasks.

Using this system also has it problems. There can easily be a tremendous gap between organization and board unless there is an effective liaison agent between them. Communication can become extremely garbled and this is about the worst thing that can happen to a center. It is often the beginning of the end.

This board may serve another function, too, particularly if it is composed of persons representing some of the center's principal referral agencies and agencies it deals with frequently. The most obvious of these agencies are the hospitals, mental health facilities, and the police. Thus the center would have a definite contact in the agency to inform said agency about the center. The representative could act as the liaison between the center and the agency. The center could give the agency feedback about its services and vice-versa. Also, when an agency makes changes in its services, it is up to the representative on the board to inform the center.

There are also centers which operate out of a specific agency, staffed by their people and/or other volunteers. One of these, "Hotline" in Los Angeles, works from the Children's Hospital. Many centers are offshoots from a county mental health clinic. Additionally, there are many programs which are church or university based. Others operate as nonprofit corporations; the process for incorporating a center is discussed in Chapter IV on funding.

Operations of RoadHouse, Colorado State University

RoadHouse, Colorado State University's center, incorporates many of these ideas. The decisions for the center are made by a three-member board. Each member has a specific responsibility in the three areas referred to earlier. They are finance, office operations-scheduling, and publicity and public relations. Unless it is felt that an issue must be voted upon by the entire membership of the organization, the board makes the decisions. Also, there is a paraprofessional, whose job it is to keep the directors informed about events occurring outside the organization which influence the organization and the people using it. The paraprofessional is a student who has had experience in RoadHouse. This position or job is the liaison between the center, the faculty advisor, and the agencies RoadHouse uses. The faculty advisor coordinates training and does some public relations work, i.e. reassuring the university community that RoadHouse has not yet become a subversive organization. She has input on suggestions for RoadHouse but ultimately, with the exception of making suggestions for parts of training program, she does not have a voice in most of the decisions that must be made. She is used in an advisory capacity for the most part.

RoadHouse also has an extensive advisory board which functions just as their title suggests—in an *advisory* capacity. These agencies include: police—university and city, medical facilities—university and city, university counseling center and the county mental health clinic, city fire department, welfare office, university housing office, academic advising office, office of student relations, the federally and city funded Drug Education Project, as well as the faculty advisor and the para-professional. This board meets approximately once every three months or when otherwise deemed necessary.

This arrangement makes available a channel of communications so that the ideas may be exchanged. Changes in the agencies will thus be known to those who need the information—specifically those who call and are referred by RoadHouse. Again, the center is able to give any agency feedback about its services and vice-versa. A good line of communication is basic to the successful operation of a center and cannot be stressed enough. Communication to and from the advisory board to the operating board to the volunteers must flow easily for a successful center operation.

OFFICE OPERATIONS AND POLICIES

Methods vary from center to center, phone-in and walk-in, but a few general ideas pertain to all centers.

1. Conversations must be kept confidential and not leave the office. The only exception to this is if you talk with a professional about a problem you have encountered.

2. When a worksheet is filled out it is not to leave the office.

3. Bulletin boards and notices must be kept up-to-date and in some semblance of order.

4. Files of information and referrals must be kept up-to-date.

5. The contents of the files shall not leave the office.

6. The office is not a place for parties. Sometimes a center will place limits on how many volunteers may be there at one time. Also, in some cases there can be no "dropping in" by the volunteers.

7. No drugs or alcohol shall be in the office. If you are not in touch with reality, you cannot expect to be able to help someone whose problems are only too real for him.

8. It is easier to work in an office when you can find things in a reasonable length of time.

9. Messages and personal calls for volunteers must be kept to a minimum. If a volunteer must make a personal call, use (if applicable) the outgoing or business line.

10. The noise level must be at a minimum when a phone rings.

Phone Operations and Policies

One of the most important things about the phone is the attitude the volunteer has when it rings. No matter what is disturbing him at the moment, or what his personal beliefs are, they can not be allowed to interfere while he is on the phone.

As for the phones themselves, it is advisable to have a hold button on them. An outgoing line (unpublished number) is a good idea also. If all the other lines are full, you will not be in a bind for a line if you have to call out, nor will you be tying up an incoming line. Also, if your service is located on campus and operates through a university switchboard, it is a good idea to have an off-campus number, too. Therefore, if anything happens to the university switchboard, you will still be able to function. Another idea is a tap-in service for conference calls. A setup whereby more than one person in the office can hear and/or respond to a caller (conference type) can be used. However, this may be a delicate subject. When do you put a call on an open line like that? It is usually up to the caller. Any of the actual phone services will have to be discussed with the phone company that serves the center. Rates and services vary from area to area. Some centers receive a very minimal phone bill.

Most, if not all, centers have the policy that when answering the phone you remain anonymous. One method of answering the phone is, for example, "RoadHouse, Sue speaking, may I help you?" In this way you have identified the center. Giving a first name also makes it easier for the caller to respond; but further personal information, full name, address, etc. should not be given out since it can turn into a bad situation. First of all, the center is not a dating service. Also, it can create problems when a caller finds your home phone number and starts calling you constantly. There are times when you might want to give a caller your home phone, but as a general rule, it can result in difficulties. This is also true in regard to leaving the center to go out and meet someone who called in on something other than an emergency. There is a greater variance between centers on this issue, though. It may also depend on who the volunteers are. In addition, some centers permit the men to go out, but not the women. Other centers discourage it completely or say it is up to the person involved.

The phone should be answered as quickly as possible. One philosophy (RoadHouse) is that if you let it ring once, the call and the volunteer can collect their thoughts. If you let it go to the third ring, the caller might think no one will answer and become anxious.

When you answer the phone and get what you might think is the strangest call imaginable, do not laugh it off or ignore it. You might *know* that it is a crank call, and it may very well be one, but treat it seriously. This does not mean you have to be morose, but the person calling might be testing you. If you handle the call as if it were a real and not a crank call, he may call back with a real problem.

There are three things that can be done when a volunteer does not know what information a caller wants. He can put the line on hold, *as briefly as possible,* and find out. He can get a phone number and call back, or he can make a referral to a person or agency who will have further information. Under most circumstances, the *caller* should terminate the call, not the *volunteer.* The caller may spend an hour beating around the bush and testing the volunteer before he gets to what is really bothering him. When a shift is under-staffed, it may be advisable to put the remaining lines on hold. A caller pouring out his heart does not appreciate being placed on "hold" and the second caller does not appreciate being asked to call back. If the lines are busy, the problem is solved. There are obvious drawbacks to this. Each center will have to formulate its own policy.

Almost all centers have some sort of worksheet to fill out about the calls or persons who use the service. This aids in general evaluation and also indicates which areas need more information or help from agencies (see Appendix A). By the way, writing legibly is a great asset. Keeping these worksheets filed in one place, file cabinet or notebook, helps for easy reference.

A policy decision is necessary regarding whether or not to accept collect or toll calls. This will vary because of your area and funds or lack of them. Also, a policy must be set as to whether or not long-distance calls may be made from the office phone.

For many centers it is impossible to staff 'round-the-clock service. If the service is not available 24 hours a day, there are many things that can be done besides just letting the phone ring during off hours. Again this is somewhat governed by the center's financial status. A tape recording can be made to inform the caller of office hours, and if desired, some of the major referral agencies and their phone numbers. It can also give the number of a person "on-call."

A person who is "on-call" is someone who takes over the service for a given number of hours when the office is not open. The calls can be taken at home or wherever he chooses. On-call personnel may be the volunteers or a professional person such as a minister, a doctor, etc. Another use for the on-call system arises when the service is open. If the volunteers run into trouble, they can contact the person who is on-call, before they panic. This works as a referral for the volunteer instead of for the caller.

Another method is the answering service. This can be more diversified than the tape recording. Again, it can give office hours and major referrals. If the phone company in your area cannot automatically switch the call over to a number of someone on-call, perhaps the answering service will be able to do so. The answering service can take messages. If you use an answering service, it is wise to call the service when the office opens and again when it closes each day. If the answering service can tap a call into someone on-call, they should find out first whether the call is for general information. If it is, the call probably should not be transferred since the volunteer would not have the information files with him and could not be of much service.

If the answering service cannot tap into a line of a person on-call, they may give out that person's number. There are pros and cons on this. Some centers use it successfully while others just cannot. The number the answering service gives out will most likely be a home phone. Part of this problem has already been discussed. Additionally, if Mrs. Smith's son answers the phone "Smith residence," the caller knows who he is talking with. In a big city it might not make any difference, as there may be seven thousand Smiths in the directory, but in a small town it may be a real problem. If the little boy does not know what a center is, or if the fact that mom is on call was not explained, or if he is too young to understand, the results to the caller could be very bad. Some people have taken care of this problem by saying that no one but he/she is to answer the phone during the time he/she is on call; and any other personal call that comes in must be kept brief. For some centers this has worked out extremely well.

Walk-in

Quite a bit of the information that applies to the phone center also applies to a walk-in center. There are differences, though. In the walk-in center, if it also functions as a phone center, there should be some separation and privacy for the phone personnel if possible. This way you do not have to worry about a tremendous noise level or having someone listening over your shoulder. In a walk-in center, the reception to anyone who walks in must be warm, but not maudlin. If a client is rather hesitant about coming in to begin with, and the volunteer is gushing with warmth and enthusiasm to help, the client might feel suffocated and so run. Also, if the center is not set up only for crisis situations but also for information, a person who comes in for information is not going to want instant empathy when he walks in the door. A happy medium is hard to find, but necessary. Since some level of privacy will be wanted by many clients, do not bring everyone in the room into the conversation. If the center does not have rooms to use for privacy, being separated from others in the same room can be difficult but not impossible. The volunteer can ignore what is going on in the rest of the center and focus on the client. Also, if the center is both phone and walk-in, not all the volunteers should be on the phone at one time. Having a pot of coffee and hot water for tea can be a bonus for both volunteer and client. Magazines and local newspapers are also a good idea.

Physical Setup

Do not publicize the location of a phone-in center. Consideration should be given to choosing a quiet out-of-the-way area. However, a location centered in the section of the public to be served is essential to a walk-in center. Easy access to the walk-in center is essential in how effectively the center can fulfill its goals.

The office itself may be simple or very complex, depending on how extensive the center is. Whether the center be only phone-in or both walk-in *and* phone, it must be at least somewhat pleasant or there will be problems. People will not want to work in unpleasant surroundings, and in a walk-in, the people who come in will not be comfortable. Particularly in a walk-in, if the clientele mainly represents the drug culture, the office should not look like a doctor's waiting room. It should not be that prim and tidy anywhere, but a drug user would probably be especially uncomfortable in such an atmosphere. Again, this varies with the clientele that the center will serve; but in most circumstances the office should be warm and have a lived-in look.

Most centers have bulletin boards of some sort, but what is on them varies tremendously. Some centers such as the one at Santa Cruz, California, the Santa Cruz Community Switchboard, have forms for each different interest area and these are written out and posted. The categories are endless. Some of them follow: (a) messages—who called, caller's number, message, who message is for, date, (b) rides, (c) crash pads and housing, (d) sale/buy, (e) lost/found, (f) jobs, (g) clothing/food, (h) current events (weekly) and entertainment, and (i) political material—general information, no party affiliation. Santa Cruz also has a *Read This* note book, in which important information is written so everyone may be aware of it. They have a list of daily jobs, for example: Monday—update the bulletin board, Tuesday—clean the office, etc. They also have mail boxes in the office for some of the staff where messages and information may be placed. Other centers have in/out boxes set up. Suggestion boxes are another common fixture. If the center does some tutoring, a blackboard helps. The center should be set up where rest rooms are available within walking distance. Another thought to be considered is who shall have keys to the center and who will lock it and unlock it.

Resources

The files will be used extensively in any center. Therefore, it is important that they be as extensive as possible and kept up-to-date. If the center is affiliated with a university, its files must contain not only university information, but also all the community information it can find and vice-versa. This information can be filed alphabetically, according to category, and/or cross-filed in regular file cabinets or notebooks (file cabinets are easier). Also, a center can use recipe boxes with file cards strictly as a referral file. It contains, alphabetically and according to category, names, addresses and phone numbers of referral sources, and is situated by all the phones. A Roll-a-Dex may be more convenient than a recipe box. Another way to keep this information is on a clipboard. A small library in the center is a great help. It may include telephone directories, dictionaries and almanacs.

Reference books such as cookbooks, legal, medical, drug, often come in handy.

Scheduling and Volunteers

When scheduling personnel, a great deal of the procedure depends on the volunteers at the center. Any number of shifts can be scheduled according to the number of hours the center is open. The volunteers may select their own schedule; they may schedule themselves as they find it convenient, and whoever is in charge of scheduling (a frustrating task) can fill in the blanks with whomever is left. There may be a fixed schedule where a volunteer works at a certain time on certain days all the time. Some centers just schedule people, giving the volunteer no option unless he trades shifts with someone. This presents the problem of getting replacements when a volunteer cannot work for some reason. The responsibility may fall back on the person who does the scheduling, or the responsibility to find his own replacement may go to the person who cannot work. The problem of what to do with Sue Jones when she never appears for work and does not find a replacement, becomes whether to let her go after two misses or ten, keep her off the phones for a certain amount of time and assigning her special work, etc. Whatever the decision—make a policy and abide by it! You will save yourselves endless aggravation.

Some centers require a certain number of hours a week or month from the volunteers. This gives some sort of control to the scheduling.

Usually there is a meeting once a month for all the volunteers. This is usually a business meeting. Some centers also incorporate in-service training at this time. This meeting may or may not be mandatory. It is usually advisable that most of the volunteers come, so they are made aware of any changes.

Publicity and Public Relations

Publicity is an important factor in the life of a center. If a center does not publicize, no one will know of its existence. One way of choosing the clientele may be by limiting the areas which the publicity will effect and the people to whom it will appeal. The wording of the publicity is also important. If you are advertising a crisis-information center, people are apt to think of you only as a last resort. The publicity possibilities are many—hand-outs, pamphlets, posters, newspapers, radio and television. Some of the advertising can be done free of charge as a public service, depending on the agencies in your area. Many centers have designed wallet-sized cards with their phone numbers printed on them. An article in a newspaper at regular intervals is definitely an asset.

Public relations (PR) is another important factor in the smooth operation of a center. If you have an advisory board (such as Road-House does), part of the battle is already won. However, you must keep up with PR. A small, well-informed speakers' bureau in your organization is helpful. They may speak about the organization, the center's purpose and activities before the local PTA, Elks Club, church organizations, etc. This is a good method for soliciting funds and support from various organizations throughout the city. Good public relations can be a governing factor in who and what agencies will most support the center.

Communications with Other Centers

There are hundreds of centers with millions of ideas. It will undoubtedly be very beneficial for everyone if some sort of communications network is established between them. There are several newsletters and lists of and about centers which are available to any service, one of the best being that of the Youth Emergency Service (YES) in the Minneapolis — St. Paul area. If you contact other services, you can get new ideas and help in solving problems.

In the spring of 1971, the National Hotline Conference was held in Monterey, California. Hundreds of centers across the United States were represented. The purpose of the conference was to get people together to discuss problems and exchange ideas. (Incidentally, the two most prominent problems were group cohesion and funding.) Part of the conference consisted of talks by some prominent individuals in the crisis center and psychology fields, such as Dr. Carl Rogers. However, for the most part, groups were formed to discuss specific problems and seek some answers. A good many people left the conference feeling that much had been accomplished. I left with many new ideas that could be used in improving RoadHouse—both in its internal structure and services to its clientele. This idea of exchanging ideas and suggestions can be a very important part of keeping a center alive. I would advise keeping informed about and attending the regional and national conferences if at all possible.

This chapter has been an attempt to cover a broad spectrum of ideas on how a center could operate. Again, the ideas reviewed here are by no means the only possibilities. Ideas may be modified or expanded according to each centers' individual needs.

REFERENCES

Training Manual. Santa Cruz Community Switchboard, Santa Cruz, California, 1970.

Taub, J.: *Operations of Roadhouse.* Fort Collins, Colorado, Colorado State University Counseling Center, 1971.

VII

GETTING IT TOGETHER: GROUP COHESION

Janet Taub

A S was mentioned in Chapter VI, the main problem besides funding the center will be that of group cohesion.

Cohesion can be defined as bringing separate entities together to form a more efficient means toward a goal. Cohesion in a center can be categorized into three areas:

1. *The ability of the staff to formulate realistic goals for the center.* Dr. Glenn C. Dildine, professor at Colorado State University, has presented in his lectures, several criteria for effective goal setting:
   a. Aimed toward meeting important shared individual needs and development, which are seen as important to everyone.
   b. Aimed toward meeting important societal organization, operation and development.
   c. Realistic in the practical situation the group faces.
   d. Clearly understood by members.
   e. Individual members have high levels of commitment to defined goals.

2. *The ability of the staff members to work together to reach established goals.* There may be many different techniques for reaching a goal. However, if these separate techniques can be placed in a workable framework where no one is being stepped on, cohesion is exemplified. An example of good cohesion is mandatory especially in a walk-in center. If the staff works well together, it portrays a good model for clients to observe.

3. The ability to perpetuate beneficial growth in the center. A cohesive group is one which is flexible in its decisions. It can discuss new ideas and methods and accept them, where applicable, into the working operations of the center. The group is amenable to change and does not remain static.

A cohesive group is a group which is mature. (For a more comprehensive account of a mature group, see the outline at the end of the chapter.)

FACTORS PERTAINING TO COHESION

There are several factors which are related to the degree of cohesion in a center. Consider some of these factors throughout the discussion.

1. One variable is that of staff size. Is the staff large or small? Is its size growing, shrinking, or remaining static?

2. Who makes up the staff? Is it a peer group or people in many different age and occupational categories?

3. The rate of staff turnover is another factor. Do staff members stay long enough to build a trust level? Or do they stay only long enough to be able to connect names with faces of a few volunteers? Is this because of the organization or is it due to other factors—occupation or the amount of time the center demands?

4. The method of training is another factor. Is it ongoing or set up for a number of specific sessions during the year? If it is set up only a few times per year, is the new group trained together or in sections?

5. Another item to consider is whether the program is doing what it set out to do. Is it fulfilling at least a few of its goals and working on others?

Most of the problems with group cohesion in a center are based on a lack of communication between directors and the general staff, between the directors themselves, and between the members of the general staff itself.

SPECIFIC PROBLEMS AND POSSIBLE SOLUTIONS

There may be condescension on the part of the experienced volunteers towards the new staff members. One of the causes for this is the training schedule. If the training is ongoing and new people are coming in all of the time, there is not a great amount of distinction between old and new. This will be somewhat reinforced because many centers, and quite rightly so, have an observational period for the first few weeks that the new staff is on the phone. If the new staff is trained in sections, there may be competition between the members from different sections. Self-seeking, or self-gratifying competition, in place of working for the organization, does not help the center greatly. If each group is given the same materials and trainers are rotated between groups, this problem will diminish in size. Also, the governing body may make an obvious distinction between old and new in the way they relate to the new people or structure the organization.

There are ways in which a center may alleviate some of these problems. If there is a period of observation when new staff begins to
work, it should be as brief as possible. Hopefully the center has obtained a majority of good people through selection, and the training
program has been successful. When the new people have gone through
selection and training processes, have been accepted to the staff, and
have gone through the period of observation, there is no reason why
they should constantly have to prove themselves. It is unfair to apply
this type of pressure.

When the list of staff members is compiled, there should not be a
distinction between old and new. The old volunteers and administration should make a conscious effort to refrain from referring to the
most recent arrivals as "new staff" as quickly as possible. The old
volunteers should not be over protective—let the new staff work. If
they need help it can be given, but do not assume duties that the
new staff is perfectly capable of handling. Also, everyone makes mistakes. Do not ride a new member into the ground for a little error.

Some staff members may feel that they could do quite a bit for the
organization, but no one seems to hear them. Because of this the staff
member may become disenchanted and drop out of the organization.
When the staff feels that they have been asking and telling things to
the directors, and feel they are being ignored, they quit talking. This
works both ways—staff to directors and directors to staff. When one
or both sides cease talking there is no communication and no growth
in the organization. The rate of dropouts will increase and maintain
at a high level.

One frequent problem is that often the directors separate themselves from the general staff. They become somewhat unapproachable.
This is often done without the realization of the directors. Do the
directors actually work in the center? Are they the only ones to make
decisions? How are the general meetings set up? Do the directors do
all the talking? How are the chairs set up? Are the directors at the
front of the room facing the rest of the staff? It has been found that
if people sit in a circle so that each person can see everyone else, communication seems to be easier. Also, the directors are then a part of
the group instead of separate from them, merely by a physical setup.

The center at the University of New Mexico, Agora, has a procedure which seems to work quite well in getting the staff to partici-

pate in the meetings and, as a carry-over, to the general operations. At the beginning of each general meeting, index cards are passed out to every staff member. Each person is asked to write something on the card—a grievance or complaint related to the organization, a compliment to someone, a joke, any comment. Then the cards are collected and discussed by the whole group. This encourages staff involvement. If there is a complaint expressed, the group can discuss it, and hopefully they will arrive at a possible solution, and find people who be willing to work at obtaining that solution. It is also a good time to suggest new ideas to the group and get some discussion and feedback on them. Once this has been done, it opens up communications and gets ideas flowing. Other problems which have come up can be discussed with a little more ease.

One thing is rather common to a general meeting: the meeting is primarily a problem-solving activity and does not usually deal with actual interpersonal skills to any great degree. There are activities with which the staff can become involved that work on these skills. Two of these might be (a) a workshop dealing with interpersonal and communication skills, and (b) a retreat where the staff takes off for a couple of days and honestly communicates what each member is feeling about the center and himself.

Another problem may arise in the form of complaints about the directors or the way they are working. This may be because the general staff does not understand what responsibilities the directors actually have. A clear statement of each job may help here. It will also help in getting some participation from the group. Many times the directors will need some help in various areas. If a member of the staff knows what the basic job entails, he may volunteer to help the director in his area. This is particularly true in such areas as public relations and publicity. It also gives the volunteer experience in the area, which helps if he/she would like to become a director.

Sometimes the service publicizes itself as one thing, but once a person becomes a staff member, he/she realizes the service is not what it is supposed to be. If a person is silent, or talks but is not heard, staff members are apt to disappear rapidly. The turnover in staff is apt to be quite high. If length of service of staff members is brief, no level of trust can be built. This affects the level of competent operation of the center.

Problems also arise when the directors make plans for change but cannot find any staff members who will be willing to help. Maybe the directors have removed themselves from the general staff too much. Maybe they have not communicated the proposed change well, or to enough staff members. Maybe the staff members who know about the change really do not care, in which case the center needs a more carefully selected staff. In any case, the directors must be sure that the staff, all of it, is aware of what is trying to be accomplished. Perhaps if there are some volunteers who might help, the work on the proposed project could be exchanged for something else. For example, if there are a required number of hours a volunteer must work at the center, this time could be used in exchange for working time in the center.

An example of the communication problem can be illustrated here. One center had a group of directors who decided that the staff should have a Christmas party. They thought it would be nice if they organized it and had the rest of the staff attend. The only people who showed up for the party were the ones who had organized it—extremely disappointing to say the least.

With a large staff there is more of an opportunity to form subgroups within the whole group. These groups form because of a variety of circumstances, i.e. friends, interest groups. These groups can be a problem because many of them will become too independent of the group as a whole. They will not be contributing to the center as a whole, but only as isolated segments. Even in a small staff there will be subgroups. However, these will be fewer than in a large group, and the separation between them may not be as large. In a small staff there are likely to be two subgroups. One of these is made of those who work at the center often and form a close circle of friends. The other is apt to be made up of those people who do not work at the center as frequently and make friends with only a limited number of other staff members. This is not necessarily detrimental to the health of the center, but the situation *can* get out of hand. With a large staff and many subgroups, it seems easier, if not checked, for these subgroups to drift farther and farther apart from one another. This can be very detrimental to the center's operations. Information is not exchanged efficiently and working conditions may become difficult.

Another factor in staff relations is who serves as the staff. If the staff is not made up of peer groups only, there may be added problems. This does *not* mean the staff should be peer group only, merely that in a diversified group there may be sensitive situations of which to be aware. Problems may result from professional people being too protective of nonprofessional people, condescension towards the younger members of the staff, and so on.

Since cohesion depends a great deal on communication, the main solution to the lack of cohesion would be communication. Just being aware of the problem does not solve it. Act on solutions; discuss suggestions; use the little "clues" that appear with various staff members. Remember that the word "thanks" goes a long way. If someone does something well, or goes out of his way to do something, do not let it go unnoticed. A reward system of *any* sort is a good idea, even if it consists of merely praising people at a general meeting.

Another idea is that of an identification card. This seems to give many people a concrete sense of belonging and often brings the group together.

If you have read this chapter and find that you need further help, try to contact a qualified person in the community with whom you may consult. If you are located near a university or college, one of your best resources will be a professor in the sociology department. If not, perhaps a member of your advisory board or someone from an agency the center uses for referrals could help. These *are* people who will help. You must *seek these people out*; they will not step forward.

The following is a checklist which the center may use to rate staff cohesion, and the areas in which the staff needs improvement.

CHARACTERISTICS OF A "MATURE" GROUP

Guidelines for Group Analysis and Participation

GLENN C. DILDINE

A. Climate of Feeling—Toward Mutual Acceptance and Trust
  1. Person-to-person interaction
    a. Increasing sensitivity to one's own feelings, and to those of others.
    b. Willingness to face one's own responsibilities, including:
      (1) Self-discipline, accepting restraints on own behavior.
      (2) Assisting others as help is needed.

c. Accepting right of other person to be different; accepting that people inevitably are different, "not necessarily like me."

2. Group climate

a. Improved ability to withstand tension, frustration, disagreement.

b. Decrease in time needed to recover from threatening group situations. Peaks and valleys of emotional group crises become less personal and threatening.

c. Feeling that the things the group is working on are also important to each other.

B. Communication below the Surface

1. Effective listening

a. Members try to hear what the other person is trying to communicate, from viewpoint of the speaker.

2. Continual feedback

a. Members check back with speaker, before responding, to test whether listener has actually received the message as the sender intended it.

C. Group Goals and Organization to Achieve Goals

1. Understanding and agreement

a. Members truly understand the various alternative goals available to the group, and the implications of each alternative.

b. Members accept the alternative chosen, so that each willingly goes along with and contributes to its achievement.

c. Members periodically check and review their chosen directions. Are they still practical and generally valued? Group will change directions and plans, if this seems appropriate.

2. Organization to accomplish goals

a. Group organizes well (establishes appropriate subcommittees; individuals accept specific contributory roles, and carry out their jobs).

b. Increased efficiency in locating problems and goals, in problem-solving and decision-making, and in mutual help as needed. Is decision-making manipulated authoritatively by one or a few, or more appropriately reached by discussion-consensus procedures?

c. Increasing tolerance and awareness that progress takes time.

D. Influence, Power and Status

1. Style of leadership

a. Increased ability for group to be self-directed, rather than dependent on leader for most ideas, decisions and action.

b. Person(s) in positions of influence and leadership (who are they?) exert their influence more toward confidence in and support for increasing *member* involvement and decision-making, rather than keeping such authority in own hands (leader).

2. Subgroup organization
   a. Existing close friendship or work subgroups are more cooperative and helpful with each other than they are either ignoring or rejecting.

NOTE: This guideline was adapted and expanded from that of Leland P. Bradford and was primarily stated as a guide to characteristics of a production group.

REFERENCES

Bradford, Leland P.: *Group Development.* Bethel, Maine National Training Laboratories, 1961.

VIII

EVALUATION: LET US DO WHAT WE SAID WE WOULD

JOHN E. HINKLE

PERHAPS the most basic question in any evaluation is, How do you know when a program or service accomplishes what it sets out to accomplish? This is certainly true of a crisis center as well as any other type of service that might be offered to a consumer group. As Ciocco (1960) said: ". . . a community agency sincerely interested in measuring the effects of its activities on the health of the people must be willing to establish a research program for this purpose." In the case of a crisis center, the consumer groups are those individuals who use the services of the center. Evaluation of the activities of a crisis center involves the impact of those program activities not only on the consumer but also on those individuals rendering the service.

It is the purpose of the evaluation to supply feedback concerning the consequences of various activities. This includes possible methods of correcting unwanted side effects resulting from a particular approach or approaches to an existing problem. Such approaches utilize program evaluation, not to be confused with people evaluation.

Frequently, program evaluation has really meant *people evaluation*. Programs are inadvertently tied to people rather than to a problem to be resolved or a goal to be achieved. If the approach to a particular problem proves ineffective, the people involved are replaced or at least chastised. This solution says nothing about an effective or ineffective *program evaluation,* as it seems easier to attribute any difficulties to the people who have been involved.

An outcome of seeing program evaluation as people evaluation without separating the two, is that good talent is not utilized because individuals do not want to risk participation in a program that is influenced by something beyond their control. Such mixing of people and program evaluation is to be avoided.

Evaluation usually deals with three basic concerns: (a) objectives of the program or activity to be evaluated, (b) the model or models to be used which will provide a framework to look at the program, and (c) statistical techniques used to understand the data gathered. There are several steps that are useful in meeting these basic concerns:

1. *Intent of program.* Questions should be formulated in such a way as to supply answers for the decision makers, i.e. Does the program serve all the people it was intended to serve? Is the program doing what it was designed to do?

2. *Useful facts and data.* The kinds of facts and other data needed to answer the questions formulated should be identified. Tests or scales constructed for the specific program, case histories, interviewing schedules and questionnaires can provide data about what is done in the program.

3. *Time and people.* It is essential at the beginning of any program to plan the amount of time to be spent in the various activities of the program. Tied closely to this is selection of the types of people to work in the program as well as specification of their duties and responsibilities.

4. *Program cost.* In any evaluation a final consideration is some estimate of the cost of the program. This is often the most important one for administrators.

Basic in any program evaluation are the program objectives. Although researchers often are included as last minute personnel in a program staff, they can be much more effective if they are included initially as the program is designed. Here, some help from a psychologist or sociologist could be most useful.

When the policies or objectives of the organization are specified and a program designed to carry out the objectives, then evaluation findings give feedback to the organization. Policies can then be modified or changed, or the programs carrying out the policies can be modified, changed, and strengthened (Suchman 1967).

One of the most difficult problems in an evaluative research is to state the objectives of a particular program in specific terms so that they can be measured. In this way you can know clearly when your program has accomplished the objectives. For example, one objective might be to have three trained people on duty at all times. Thus, after training it should be easy to demonstrate that three people who had completed the program are on duty. This might be demonstrated through the use of a log book where trained staff sign in and out.

A crisis center should have as its first and foremost purpose, the saving of lives. A second objective should be to deal with individuals at times of crisis. A third objective could be to suggest referrals to other agencies who can provide help for the individual in order to reduce his inability to deal with crises in the future. In keeping with these objectives, a crisis center can, through evaluation, demonstrate that it plays an important part in the health and well-being of the community members and thus should be supported by the community (Parad 1965).

Four functions usually found in a crisis center are:

1. Helping people recognize their problems and providing alternatives to possibly resolve the concern.
2. Referrals to appropriate agencies and/or persons within the community for further information or help.
3. Giving information about available community services.
4. Continuous training for staff performing the service.

In light of the above discussion on evaluation and the four functions of a crisis center, the following procedures, modified from Stake (1969), are suggested as an evaluation framework.

Section 1: Objectives of the evaluation. Included here are answers to such questions as, Does the center provide the service it set out to provide, Who knows if the center does what it set out to do, What decisions about the center need to be made, and Based on evaluation of objectives, are changes in order?

In looking at the evaluation objectives of a crisis service, the consumer to be served by the center is, of course, important. Equally important are the people to be served by the evaluation of the crisis service. This latter group are the individuals who are going to be concerned with continuing the service, those individuals who may wish to set up a similar service and significant other individuals in the community. In this latter group would fall administrators of funds to be used in continued support of the service.

It is important to state specifically the content of a program for a crisis center. This refers to the kinds and availability of services to be offered and the limitations under which such services may operate. For example, if professional services are to be immediately available on a walk-in basis, then extensive medical and psychiatric resources are needed. If the center offers an information-only type of service or sympathetic listening by trained paraprofessionals, then more limited resources such as professionals on call might be more appropriate.

Section 2: Specifics of the program. Does the content of the program reflect its philosophy to help, i.e. is the program helping people in crisis? Are people in the community using the program?

Some measure of the use of the program by the consumer could be obtained from other agencies within the community. For example, if referrals to such agencies as the welfare department, city police, ministers, physicians, and other health services come from the crisis center, then knowledge of the use of those agencies by community members could be made. Periodic assessment of knowledge of the service, once it is established by personnel in other agencies and/or individuals rendering service to the public could be gathered. This same information could be gathered from the private sector, i.e. physicians, psychologists, ministers, etc.

In evaluating the use of the crisis center, knowledge should be obtained about the consumer and the kinds of concerns he has. For example, a structured tally sheet completed by those staff members who are giving the service is a useful approach. This could be gathered at specific, regular intervals. The tally sheet would simply be a listing of the concern or kinds of crisis expressed by the individual utilizing the services of the crisis center. This information could include where he lives, family and work, status, etc., and then be compared with demographic data about individuals in the community, their family size, education, and socioeconomic level. Distance factors (e.g. how far needed to travel to the center) could also be assessed. Such information would be important in making such modification in the program as location of the crisis center and the kinds of information about the service to be presented to the community.

Section 3: Program outcomes. What kinds of experiences do the people have who work in the program, and are the experiences used to improve the program? Also, do the consumers of the service like or dislike the program and why? What kind of side effects, both good and bad, occur?

In evaluation of a crisis center, it is necessary to keep in mind that no service evaluation can be complete without taking into account the preferences and priorities of all the groups of people who may benefit or be injured by the service. Included are those individuals providing the service as well as those on the receiving end of such a service. For example, the individual giving the service can become more knowledgeable about the community in which he lives. He may become more effective in communicating with other individuals he sees in the state of crisis.

With the names of the individuals obtained at the crisis center, follow-up in terms of consumer satisfaction could be obtained through direct survey of users of the service. Knowledge about and value placed on provision of such a service in the community obtained by surveyer from both users and nonusers of the service, could be good information to obtain. Such information would not only tap consumer's use of the program but also determine the consumers gain or loss from having used the services offered.

Still other knowledge of the programs' effect in the community can be made after the service has been in operation over a number of months' time. Here, one would look at both positive and negative comments about the service from other agencies. This information would be about individuals who had received service from the crisis center and then referred to other local community resources. Such questions as, Was the referral appropriate, Was it effective in life problem of the individual, Was the information given to the individual about the agency by the crisis center accurate, could be used to obtain knowledge of the centers' effect in the community.

Evaluation questionnaires given to the agency people every three months might be a basic way of gathering other data about the service. Such questionnaires could include rating scales and open-ended questions for suggested changes or modifications in the program. This information could then be given to the staff of the crisis center so that modifications in the program could be made, if the staff thought such changes were appropriate.

Assessment should be made of other changes occurring in those people who provide the service. For example, does such an individual become more involved with what goes on in his community? Does he take part in other community activities, more so than before his experience in working in a crisis center? Another important question is, Does he become more effective in interpersonal relationships? For example, did he learn some techniques of interpersonal skills that provide him with more satisfactory interpersonal relationships, not only in terms of his work, but in his family and day-to-day living. Experience suggests that when individuals are trained to deal with crises, they become more effective in other aspects of their lives, not only on the basis of the knowledge but in terms of the kinds of experiences they have in helping other human beings. Structured self-reports and reports of activities could be used to get this information.

Section 4: Judgment of worth. Did the program work; is it useful to the community? Is the program effective in reaching its objectives, does it cost too much or is it low-cost relative to the number of people served?

Perhaps one of the most difficult issues to deal with is the usefulness of a service to the community. The losses or negative effects occurring to both consumers and the staff involved in such a crisis center is an important part of the question of usefulness. Essentially, this is evaluation of the failure rate of the program, both in terms of the inability to meet the objectives as far as the consumer is concerned, and the inability to train the staff effectively. In the latter case, continually modifying the training programs in light of feedback from the participants would be highly desirable. Such feedback can be gained in terms of difficulties reported by those trained and suggestions they may have for additional information needed in the program. Staff personality and selection procedures are important here. The selection criteria of the kind of individual needed to function effectively in a crisis center should be decided beforehand. Here professional consultation to spell out criteria can be most helpful.

As to negative impact on the consumer, this is a more difficult area to evaluate. One possibility is a monthly newsletter sent to all individuals and agencies who have had contact with the center eliciting particularly the crisicisms of, and suggestions for, improvement in the service. To systematically evaluate the impact of a crisis center, frequency counts of crisis situations could be obtained from other agencies and private individuals in the community before establishing the center. After the establishment of the crisis center, the same data can be periodically gathered. One might find that individuals and agencies rendering service to individuals would see fewer crises occurring in their practice after the establishment of such a center.

Another indicator of the worth of the program is the cost in dollars to the community that supports the crisis program. Evaluation in this area should involve a long-term approach, with different kinds of questions to be asked at different intervals as the program operates. Such questions might include the efficiency of this manner of dealing with community crisis. The need for expanded staff or curtailed staff in the crisis center in terms of workload can be made by a tally of number of people served per staff member. The number of professionals involved and the cost of their time by means of records of hours spent can be helpful cost information.

The continuing functioning of a crisis center program rests to a great extent on the kind of evaluation information discussed above. In addition, decisions about modifications in the program are usually made on the basis of how the program is functioning and the kinds of data that are utilized to assess the service.

This way of asking questions and organizing the information gathered is one approach to evaluating a crisis center. Although several complex evaluation models could be utilized to evaluate such a program, often a more simplified approach like the one suggested may be the best.

REFERENCES

Ciocco, A.: On indicies for the appraisal of health department activities. *Journal of Chronic Diseases, 11:*521, 1960.

Parad, H. J. (Ed.): *Crisis Intervention: Selected Readings.* New York, Family Service Association of America, 1965.

Stake, R. E.: Evaluation design, instrumentation, data collection and analysis of data. *Educational Evaluation.* Columbus, Ohio, State Superintendent of Public Instruction, 1969, pp. 58-71.

Suchmas, E. A.: *Evaluative Research: Principles and Practices in Public Service and Social Action Programs.* New York, Russell Sage Foundation, 1967.

IX

DRUGS: THE ROLE OF THE CRISIS CENTER

MARV MOORE

CRISIS centers receive frequent requests for accurate drug information, as well as for assistance with drug-related problems and crises. The success of a crisis center depends on volunteers who have been systematically trained to deal with these requests. The purpose of this chapter is to define the essential topics and skills that must comprise the training of crisis center volunteers for handling such requests for help. These topics include (a) who uses drugs and why, (b) knowledge of the commonly used drugs and their effects, (c) how to competently handle typical drug-related crises, and (d) the crisis center's policy on drug usage and abuse. The chapter concludes with some suggestions for integrating these topics into an effective training process.

WHO USES DRUGS

The first question to address is Who uses drugs? In contemplating this question, it helps to think of drugs in a broader sense, as "mood-altering agents," (Dohner, 1970) and rephase the question: Who in our culture uses mood-altering agents? If the reader will scan the list below of commonly-used mood-altering agents (Dohner, p. 2), a list not meant to be inclusive, he will see for himself the extensive range of such elements.

Mood-altering Agents

alcohol	marijuana, hashish	methadone
amphetamines	barbiturates	morning glory seeds
antihistamines	bromides	opium, heroin
aspirin	caffeine	peyote, mescaline
banana skins	cocaine	STP
food	cough syrup	tobacco
glue	Darvon®	tranquilizers (prescribed)
laxatives	ephedrine	tranquilizers (not prescribed)
LSD	ether	vitamins

Obviously, the ingestion of mood-altering agents escapes no age group or social class. The reader probably recognized in the list his own favorite relaxant or stimulant.

Drug usage, as regularly encountered by a crisis center, is not confined solely to experimenting or disturbed adolescents. The crisis center volunteer will render more effective assistance to all callers if he remembers this fact. Although adolescents ingest their drugs with the loudest bravado, Americans from all age groups depend heavily on mood-altering agents to maintain their health and sense of mental well-being.

A second way to approach the question of who uses drugs is to consider how frequently a person uses a given mood-altering agent. A mistake made by unknowledgeable people is to lump all persons into two categories, users and non-users. This over-simplification eliminates important differences between drug users which a crisis center volunteer must, as a matter of course, understand. There are *at least* the following subgroups of drug users.

1. *Non-users* themselves consist of three subgroups: persons clearly against drug usage, persons who do not care one way or the other, and persons interested in the phenomenon of drug usage but undecided as to whether they will use drugs in the near future. Non-users are likely to call a crisis center primarily on behalf of another (e.g. a parent frightened by the discovery of her son's "pot" smoking).

2. *Active contemplators* are those persons seriously thinking about experimenting with one mood-altering agent or another. They are very apt to call a crisis center seeking accurate drug information or assistance in reaching a feasible decision.

3. The *just-tried* group are persons who have just had their first drug experience or experiences. Their feelings about the experience may range from being very scared or confused to joyous and anxious to share the good news with another. Members of this group, disturbed by or in the middle of an unpleasant "trip," are not uncommon callers.

4. *Occasional users* are persons who use one drug or another infrequently for purposes of relaxation, self-exploration, or enhancing certain interpersonal experiences. Occasional users seldom call a crisis center since their drug usage is usually integrated into a functioning pattern of competent living.

5. *Regular, reasonably frequent users* consist of those persons who, at least for the present, see drug usage as a major aspect of successful living. Some members of this group would say they are part of a "counter-culture" where drugs play an integral part in building a sense of community, in exploring oneself, in enhancing the experience of living, or as a religious experience. Although middle and lower class Americans may see these persons as immature and/or lazy, regular users would probably contend that they are functioning more than adequately in their own simpler and less competitive "society." Quite naturally, the regular users seldom, if ever, seek assistance from a crisis center, especially since they tend to trust only each other with personal crises and "bum trips."

6. *Heavy, chronic users* are those persons who have become physically or psychologically dependent upon the drug they are using. Adolescents addicted to heroin or psychologically dependent on Methedrine® ("speed") are likely to seek help from a crisis center only under two conditions: (a) if there is in the community an established treatment program for such users (e.g. a methadone treatment program for heroin addicts) and (b) under the most severe of crises such as contemplated suicide, when no friend can be reached. Persons addicted to and/or dependent on barbiturates are most likely to call, especially during the crisis of contemplated or attempted suicide.

It is important that crisis center volunteers be aware of the difference between all categories of drug users, and that they employ their knowledge of such differences as guidelines for treating each person as a unique individual with his own special problem.

WHY DO PEOPLE USE MOOD-ALTERING AGENTS

The second question that crisis center volunteers need to grapple with is, Why do people use mood-altering agents anyway? The volunteer in training will find Dr. Dohner's paper, *Mood-altering Agents in American Society: Why?* (1970), required reading for understanding this complex question. Dr. Dohner presents over a dozen different reasons why Americans employ mood-altering agents. An obvious reason for using drugs is to decrease or eliminate physical pain or discomfort. Other physically-oriented reasons for usage are to avoid fatigue and to assist in dieting. Many persons find drugs an easy means to relaxation and recreation; witness the social drinker who loosens up at the Friday night party. Still others are curious and desire a new experience. Several reasons for using mood-altering agents are self-destructive and clearly depress psychological growth. Some drugs afford an effective escape from the boredom or excessive anxiety of an unproductive or meaningless life, or from just the normal anxiety necessary to meet the daily expectations of living. Still other drugs are ingested or injected to reduce the anxiety of intimacy required for significant human relationships. Some adolescents find the danger involved with certain drugs an irresistible lure; peer pressure may support or deter such dangerous experimentation. On the other hand, the escape form of drug usage may also reflect an attempt to establish an independent identity, an attempt at self-discovery through the resolution of adolescent rebellion and rejection of parental or societal values. For the poor and racially discriminated against, drugs may represent a bearable solution to a continuously unacceptable and rejecting environment. Among the potentially positive uses of drugs is the enhancement of creativity claimed by several authors and artists. Finally, there are those individuals who sincerely believe certain drug-induced states to be mystical-religious experiences.

In reading the above paragraph the reader will note that there are motives for drug usage which are potentially both constructive and destructive for human growth. People use drugs for both good and bad reasons! Armed with this knowledge, the crisis center volunteer increases his effectiveness by believing and exploring with those seeking help, especially adolescents, the healthy reasons for drug usage as well as the less healthy ones.

COMMONLY USED DRUGS

There is a basic body of knowledge concerning the commonly used mood-altering agents with which every crisis center volunteer needs to be thoroughly familiar. The broadest groups of commonly used drugs are the narcotics (opiates), the depressants (sedatives and hypnotics), stimulants, hallucinogens, and marijuana. For each of the drugs within each of these broad groups, crisis center staff need to study at least the following:

1. Slang names for each drug.
2. Usual single dosage taken.
3. Short-range physical and psychological effects.
4. Long-range physical and psychological effects.

5. Dangers inherent in usage.
6. Alleged and real benefits to the user.
7. Immediate effects and symptoms of overdosage.

It is recommended that each volunteer be given a copy of Joel Fort's "Comparison Chart of Major Substances Used for Mind Alteration" (Fort, 1969) for regular work reference. Fort's chart presents in a convenient two-page form a summary of answers to most of the seven questions above.

Crisis centers will also want to secure for their reference libraries all of the following publications:

1. Dependence on cannabis (marijuana). Reprint from *The Journal of the American Medical Association, 201:*368-371, 1967.
2. Dependence of LSD and other hallucinogenic drugs. Reprint from *The Journal of the American Medical Association, 202:*47-50, 1967.
3. Dependence on amphetamines and other stimulant drugs. Reprint from *The Journal of the American Medical Association, 197:*1023-1027, 1966.
4. Dependence on barbiturates and other sedative drugs. Reprint from *The Journal of the American Medical Association, 193:*673-677, 1965.
5. Solursh, L., and Clement, W.: Haellucinogenic drug abuse: manifestations and management. *The Canadian Medical Association Journal, 98:*407-410, 1968.
6. Coles, R., Breuner, J., and Meagher, D.: *Drugs and Youth: Medical, Psychiatric and Legal Facts.* New York, Liveright, 1970.

TYPICAL DRUG-RELATED CALLS

There are four common requests for help that crisis center volunteers must be trained to handle: (a) straightforward requests for information about a given drug or potential referral source; (b) requests where the caller seeks help in evaluating a personal decision concerning drug usage; (c) requests for crisis assistance due to an overdose of some drug or to a "bum trip"; and (d) requests from concerned parents (often scared) who have just discovered their adolescent son or daughter to be using one drug or another. Each of these typical requests merit separate discussion.

Information Requests

Persons asking for information are the simplest to aid. If an individual wishes to know something about a given mood-altering agent or where in the community to get help for a specific problem, then the volunteer should cheerfully speak forth if he has that information. If the volunteer cannot give the needed information, he should refer the person to someone or some agency who most certainly does have it, or he may quickly run down the needed fact and call the person back. It is important to remember that "information seekers" usually know what they want and do not need lectures or unsolicited help.

Decision-making Assistance

It is not unusual to receive requests to help evaluate a personal decision concerning drug usage, a decision being contemplated or one that has been recently carried out. In this situation there are two immediate temptations to which the volunteer may unwisely succumb. First, the person may phrase his plea in such a manner that he almost demands from the helper a directive for quick action. As a general rule it is best to refrain from giving such directives. Such a helpee has mixed feelings about his decision or he would not be seeking assistance in the first place, and he therefore profits from examining the pros and cons of his dilemma. The second temptation is for the helper to be seduced by the helpee into giving his own personal beliefs about drug usage. It is unwise to be seduced in this manner, for adding the helper's beliefs to the discussion usually has one of two results. It may allow the helpee to borrow an immediate solution which only delays his reaching an independent solution with which he can live, or it may make the problem-solving process more difficult because he must now contend with how he thinks the helper will react if he rejects his beliefs. Another word about the volunteer's personal biases: if the volunteer believes so strongly that a certain behavior is wrong that he cannot allow the caller to arrive at a contrary position, then that volunteer should respectfully refer the caller to a peer who is not so disposed.

In assisting the confused decision maker, the author has found the following stepwise approach to be helpful.

Step 1. The helper asks the person to be as specific as possible in answering this question, What is it that you want(ed) to accomplish by the experience? Listen and firmly encourage the person to stay with this question until he can state an expected goal for his behavior.

Step 2. Next ask the person, How would you know if your goal had been accomplished (e.g. "What specifically would you be saying and doing with whom, and when, if dropping acid helped improve your communication with people?"). Many persons rarely answer this question about their personal goals, so they find it difficult to feel either a sense of failure or accomplishment; instead, they become confused and more indecisive.

Step 3. Next ask, What things do you really know and need to know about the drug's effects to help you make your decision? Here the helper again firmly but gently guides the helpee to examine both the constructive and destructive effects that are available about the drug. Informational gaps in the person's experience are often filled by the volunteer himself, or the volunteer refers the individual to appropriate sources where the needed facts may be found.

Step 4. The next question should be, Are there any alternative means that you know for accomplishing your goals? Many persons know of specific alternatives; many others need alternatives suggested to them by the helper (e.g. "Have you thought about joining the Communication Skills Workshop at the Counseling Center to improve your interpersonal skills?").

Step 5. An inquiry with a new focus, Are you aware of the law in regard to using this particular drug? Volunteers need to know well the federal and state drug laws to be of assistance here.

Step 6. You have finished a helpful encounter. If your helpee has not solidified his decision by this time, wish him luck, and invite him to call or come back and share with you how things work out. Of course, it is possible that after your skillful assistance the person still plans to go ahead with a clearly self-destructive act and he has told you as much. *Then tell him how you feel about that!* You have earned the right to do so by proficiently completing Steps 1 through 5 (e.g. "If I could do anything about it, I'd try to stop you from experimenting with heroin.")

Concerned Parents

On occasion a crisis center receives a request for help from a concerned parent who has just learned that his adolescent is using one or more drugs. Parents who call or come in are almost always frightened or angry, or both, and their intense feelings inhibit them from knowing what to do. Therefore, the volunteer does well to first communicate to the distraught parent that he hears accurately how he feels and then to encourage him to expand and elaborate upon those feelings (e.g. "Right now you're so scared and angry you're not sure what to do next."). Second, after the parent has had sufficient time to state his initial feelings, ask him how he found out about the alleged drug usage. Often the anxious parent has inferred the worst possible outcome from the weakest of evidence. So the helper may suggest to the parent that he systematically check out his suspicions, and help him plan how to do so before he decides what action is appropriate. Third, if he has not already done so, the helper will suggest that the upset parent discuss the whole situation with the other parent before talking to his son or daughter. Deciding when and how the parent wishes to confront his son or daughter is the next important issue. The author finds it helpful to ask the helpee to imagine both parents and the adolescent in the confrontation scene (e.g. "Try to imagine what you will say and what your son's reactions will be."). Requiring the parent to imagine several alternative sequences of parent-adolescent dialogue helps him evaluate beforehand what is likely to be most and least effective. Subtle coaching and questioning of the parent in the preconfrontation imagery is necessary. Angry, over-restrictive parents need to be cautioned not to overreact; passive, "wishy-washy" parents need to be encouraged to be more openly angry and assertive in their confrontation. Finally, the volunteer will suggest the next most logical place to seek additional help if the parent-adolescent confrontation does not help the parents decide upon what to do (e.g. "You may wish to make an appointment with a professional at the Family Services Agency if things don't sort themselves out over the next few days; let me tell you how to go about that.").

Drug Crises

Crisis center staff need a working knowledge of how to deal with two types of drug crises. The first possible crisis is one where an individual has taken an overdose of some drug (barbiturates, opiates, or alcohol in combination with a barbiturate or amphetamine) which necessitates immediate medical attention. When someone contacts the crisis center by telephone concerning such a crisis the procedures to follow are as follows (*Training Manual*, 1971):

1. When the person is *unconscious*, the volunteer will need to call the Fire Department Resuscitation Squad or the appropriate emergency service in your community. Get the address, phone number and name

of the person calling along with specific directions for getting to the place where the individual is overdosed.

2. When the person is *conscious* the volunteer will need to find out:
   a. *What* the person has taken
   b. *How* it was administered (orally or otherwise)
   c. *Quantity* of the drug taken
   d. *Time elapsed* since the drug entered the body
   e. *Other drugs* taken at the same time (like alcohol)
   f. *Body weight* and *age*
   g. *Vital signs* (pulse and respiration should be checked)
   h. *Address, phone number, name, and directions to place* the call is made from

Next the volunteer calls the appropriate emergency service or ambulance and talks to the caller while waiting for aid to arrive. The helper should advise against taking any further drugs. If barbiturates, heroin, or tranquilizers have been ingested, the volunteer will firmly insist that the caller stay awake by telling him to stand up and move around, or , by getting a friend of the caller to do the same.

When the caller or friend of the caller is afraid to accept medical aid, the volunteer will have to reassure the person that the chances of legal repercussions are slim or nonexistant. Finally, if the caller refuses aid the volunteer has to make the important decision whether or not to send aid anyway. The author feels that in the case of such emergencies that it is safest to err in the direction of taking action to safeguard the caller's life.

If the individual who has taken an overdose comes into the crisis center for help the emergency procedures are the same.

Basically, the best way to handle a bad trip is whenever possible to turn it into a good trip without chemical intervention (Maclean, 1971). When a person on a bad trip calls or comes into the crisis center the first job is to provide assurance and certainty to the person that he will get immediate assistance. During the first few minutes of the conversation the helper will also attempt to find out what drug the person has taken, how he took it and how much he has taken, and how much time has elapsed since the drug entered the body. Talking down a bad trip sometimes takes several hours, and how those hours are spent depends on whether a crisis center is operating as a call-in-only agency or a drop-in agency as well.

In a call-in-only agency the volunteer cannot tie up the phone for several hours, so he chooses among several alternatives. If the caller is alone, then the volunteer may spend from a half-hour to an hour on the phone calming him down, give the person some concrete things to do to ride out the remaining hours, and call him back every hour to reassure him that the end is in sight. If friends are with the caller or easily accessible, the volunteer may teach one of them how to talk the tripper down and instruct the friend to call back if difficulties are encountered. If trained bad trip teams are available in the community or as part of the crisis center, such assistance may be solicited. The volunteer keeps the tripping caller on the phone until the bad trip team arrives.

In a drop-in center a volunteer expects to occasionally spend several hours with persons who come in experiencing a bad trip. All the same, he uses the bad tripper's friends or a bad trip team to assist him whenever possible. The procedures described so far for talking down a bad trip are the same on the phone or face-to-face.

Regardless of whether one or several hours are spent with a bad tripper, there are several helping principles that a crisis center staff should thoroughly know and practice. These principles derive from *Talking a Bad Tripper Down—Not Talking Down to a Bad Tripper* (Maclean, 1971), and are listed below with concrete examples of exactly what may be said to the tripper to make his comments effective.

Helping Principle	*Examples of Comments and Conduct*
Reduce or avoid anxiety	"You're *not* going crazy, it's the drug." (repeat often.)
	"Things are going to be strange for a while but it will wear off in about _____ hours." (estimate time based on the signs he shows and what he thinks he took . . . don't lie).
	Forewarn the tripper of effects that are likely to occur later.
	Be calm yourself. If you are uptight, he will be more so.
	Hospital emergency rooms, with their sights, aura, and smells, can scare the tripper and reinforce fears that he really is sick or crazy. Less institutional settings are more conducive to a talkdown.

Build trust

"I'd like to stay here with you until it's over."

"I want to help you turn it into a good trip."

"It's OK to talk about it, it's confidential and no one will bother us" (if that's true).

"My name is _____, I'm a *(your expertise)*, you're at *(place)*, your friends _____ and _____ are here."

Let the tripper know that you understand what he's feeling. "It must be really scary when the walls seem to move, but it's the drug doing it; I'll be with you, it'll be OK."

Avoid extraneous stimuli

Keep it quiet. Remove the phone, reroute people traffic.

Keep it darkened, turn down the lights.

Keep it friendly, tripper's friends provide warmth and the orientation base he needs.

Avoid rapid movement. Insure privacy.

Keep it here and now; help him be in control

"See this is your hand, make a fist, see you can control it."

"Breathe through your stomach, see it rise and fall, you make it move."

Anticipate his body needs (e.g. going to the bathroom, taking off his hot clothes, eating).

Keep in touch

"Here, hold onto my arm" or hold the tripper.

"Can you talk about what's going on right now?" If he starts getting panicked, change the topic; be assertive.

"A bad trip is like a raging river, you can't stop it right away, so just sit back and watch it like you would a movie."

Things to avoid   Don't be judgmental. (e.g. "It is really dumb
                         to have taken the drug.")

                         Don't play Freud. It's not the time, place, nor
                         is it the tripper's immediate need, even though
                         it may be yours.

For those few instances when talking-down techniques do not calm
an uncontrollably terrified tripper, medical assistance should be
sought. A physician or psychiatrist should be on call to back up the
crisis center staff in those rare situations when chemical control is
necessary to calm a bad trip.

Referral Sources

The benefit of a crisis center to the community depends heavily on
continuous good relationships between the center and all its available
referral sources. Personal contacts must be made with responsible
persons in each referral agency in order to secure its cooperation with
the crisis center's operations. A referral source is most likely to give its
sanction and assistance to a crisis service that is competently and systematically conceived and administered.

A manual of referral agencies should be compiled which describes
in some detail the treatment objectives and eligible patients for each
cooperating agency, the admittance procedures for eligible persons,
the phone number and address of the service, the hours during which
the service is offered, and whom to contact for further information.
To adequately handle drug crises the referral source manual should
include at least the following services:

1. Ambulance and resuscitation services
2. Local hospitals, especially emergency room procedures
3. Psychiatric services (private and public mental health clinics and
   hospitals, as well as individual practitioners)
4. The police department
5. Drug treatment and educational agencies such as methadone or alcohol treatment centers
6. Paraprofessional teams dealing with bad trips or other emergencies

Policy on Drugs

A crisis center is responsible for the physical and mental health of
its helpees. A crisis center is equally responsible for the well-being of

the public agency or institution with whom it is associated or represents. Therefore, since the ingestion of many drugs is illegal, a crisis center *must* have a clearly defined *policy on drugs*—for the simultaneous protection of helpees and agency alike. The following policy is offered as a model upon which the operation of a crisis center may be founded:

> All crisis center staff are accurately informed as to which drugs are illegal to possess or sell. The center will not intentionally aid or abet the breaking of any local, state or federal laws. Neither will the center pretend to or attempt to protect callers from the consequences of illegal acts.
>
> The crisis center will do everything in its power to help persons requesting drug information and/or assistance with drug problems or crises. Persons requesting such help will receive it in a confidential manner. No information as to their identity, use, consumption, constituents, or place of use will be provided to college administrators or to local, state, or federal narcotics agents.

The model policy above states the "persons requesting help will receive it in a confidential manner." In some states the records of a crisis center can be subpoened as evidence into court. Where this is the case, a center may protect itself by keeping records that do not reveal the identity of individual callers. Legal consultation may be necessary to insure that record keeping does, indeed, safeguard the helpee's confidentiality.

Such a policy statement should be included in brochures and public announcements of the center's operations. Likewise, the policy on drugs should be conspicuously posted on the center's premises, as a silent reminder to staff of their ethical responsibilities. Some crisis centers have also found it advantageous to post this directive: "The use of mood-altering agents other than tobacco, coffee, and tea while on the job is prohibited."

The Training Process

A training program that teaches crisis center staff to deal effectively with drug-related requests for help integrates the topics discussed in this chapter in four interlocking phases. First, trainees need to acquire the basic information necessary to function competently in the crisis agency. Paired below are the essential informational areas and suggested professionals most appropriate to make the training presentation about that area:

Informational Area	Lecturer-Presenter
1. Who uses drugs and why?	Mental health professional
2. What are the commonly used drugs and their effects and the medical management of drug crisis?	Physician or psychiatrist
3. Handling drug-related calls and crises	Mental health professional
4. Description of referral sources	Agency representatives or experienced crisis center staff member
5. Crisis center's drug policy	Experienced crisis center staff member

Organized handouts should accompany each presentation for the volunteer's fingertip reference.

In the second phase of training, professionals or experienced staff members demonstrate for the trainees how to handle the typical crisis center request for help, essentially those situations described in this chapter. The demonstration models of effective helping may be audio or video tapes or live situations involving a helper and helpee. Presentation of effective models depicting crisis management skills should precede the trainee's actual practicing of those skills.

The third phase of training consists of the trainees practicing themselves the essential skills necessary to function in the crisis center. Skill practice takes the form of trainees simulating the usual situations encountered and learning to play the roles of both helper and helpee. Experienced staff members or professional advisors give ongoing feedback to the neophyte helpers and judge when each volunteer has attained an acceptable level of competence.

Phase four involves ongoing supervision and monitoring of volunteers after they have successfully completed the initial training program. An effective crisis center is one that provides continuous feedback and supervision to *all* levels of staff members about their performance in crisis management skills. One method for achieving this is to employ the most experienced volunteers in some regular fashion to give feedback to the newest volunteers about their work. A regular supervision session (say once a month) directed by a professional or experienced staff member is necessary to provide a forum for volunteers' continuous improvement of their skills. A case presentation format where volunteers present actual crises that proved difficult to manage affords new material for role-playing practice. Assessing and enhancing volunteers' skills on a continuing basis creates a crisis center of the highest quality.

REFERENCES

Coles, R., Breuner, J., and Meagher, D.: *Drugs and Youth: Medical, Psychiatric and Legal Facts.* New York, Liveright, 1970.

Dependence on barbiturates and other sedative drugs. Reprint from the *Journal of the American Medical Association, 193*:673-677, 1965.

Dependence on amphetamines and other stimulant drugs. Reprint from the *Journal of the American Medical Association, 197*:1023-1027, 1966.

Dependence of LSD and other hallucinogenic drugs. Reprint from the *Journal of the American Medical Association, 202*:47-50, 1967.

Dependence on cannabis (marijuana). Reprint from the *Journal of the American Medical Association, 201*:368-371, 1967.

Dohner, A. B.: Mood Altering Agents in American Society: Why? Reprint of speech given to the Larimer Country Mental Health Association, Fort Collins, Colorado, January, 1970.

Fort, J.: *The Pleasure Seekers: the Drug Crisis, Youth, and Society.* New York, Grove Press, pp. 236-243, 1969.

Maclean, C.: *Talking a Bad Tripper Down—Not Talking Down to a Bad Tripper.* Training handout distributed by the Fort Collins, Colorado Drug Education Project, December, 1971.

Solursh, L., and Clement, W.: Hallucinogenic drug abuse: manifestations and management. *Canadian Medical Association Journal, 98*:407-410, 1968.

Training Manual for Volunteers. The Open Door Clinic, 5012 Roosevelt Avenue, NE, Seattle, Washington, April, 1971.

TECHNIQUES IN CRISIS INTERVENTION: A TRAINING MANUAL

NORMAN L. FARBEROW, SAMUEL M. HEILIG AND ROBERT E. LITMAN

TELEPHONE EVALUATION AND EMERGENCY MANAGEMENT OF SUICIDAL PERSONS

S UICIDE is one of the most difficult problems confronting persons in the helping professions. This applies not only to the professional therapist but to all the occupations concerned with health and well-being of the public. It is rare that any psychiatrist, psychologist, social worker, nurse, physician, clergyman, policeman or educator can conduct his affairs without at some time being faced with the need to evaluate and handle a suicidal situation.

Defining Suicide

Confusion often accompanies the use of the term *suicide*. One result of this confusion is the indiscriminate application of the term *suicidal* to patients with the implication that all such persons are in equal lethal danger. Experience has shown that suicidal persons vary in lethal potentiality from minimal to highly serious, and that each person requires individual, careful evaluation. Suicide is an ambiguous concept leading to confusions of behavior, end-result, and intention. When a person is called suicidal, these aspects must be clarified.

Characteristics of the Suicidal Situation

Crisis

The suicidal person is usually in the midst of crisis. Crisis has been defined by Webster as a "turning point in the course of a situation,"

NOTE: This chapter was originally printed as a pamphlet by the Suicide Prevention Center, Los Angeles, California, December, 1968.

and "a situation whose outcome decides whether possible bad consequences will follow." Gerald Caplan has defined crisis as a "disorganization of homeostasis (when faced with a problem) . . . which cannot be solved quickly by the individual's normal range of problem-solving mechanisms." For the person in a suicidal crisis, the principal factors are the overwhelming importance of an intolerable problem and the feelings of hopelessness and helplessness. The pressure of these feelings force him toward some actions for immediate resolution. These actions may be maladaptive, as in suicide attempts.

Crisis provides an unusual opportunity for therapeutic intervention. Crisis, by definition, implies a state that cannot be tolerated indefinitely. Something must change. The initiation and timing of therapeutic efforts during the crisis can influence the situation toward a favorable outcome.

Ambivalence

One of the features characterizing the suicidal person is ambivalence, expressed through feelings of wanting to die and wanting to live, both occurring at the same time. An example of ambivalence is the person who is angry at a love object over a real or imaginary hurt and is filled with strong feelings of both love and hate for the other. Such a person may ingest a lethal dose of barbiturates and then call someone for rescue before he loses consciousness. The relationship and strength of the two opposing impulses to live and to die will vary for different persons, and also within the same person under different conditions. Most people have a stronger wish to live than to die. It is this ambivalence which makes suicide prevention possible. In working with a suicidal person it is necessary to evaluate both motives and their relationship to each other and to ally oneself on the side of the fluctuating wish to live.

Communication

Suicidal activity is frequently a desperate method of expressing feelings of hopelessness and helplessness. Suicidal people are reduced to this method when they feel unable to cope with a problem and feel that others are not perceiving or responding to their need for help. The suicidal behavior thus becomes a claim for the attention which they feel they have lost. The communication may be in terms of verbal statements such as "I no longer want to live" or "I am going to kill myself"; or it may be in terms of actions such as the procuring fo pills or guns, a sudden decision to prepare a will, or the giving away of treasured possessions. The communication may also be either direct or indirect and is frequently aimed at a specific person. When it is indirect the problem is to recognize the intent of the disguised message and to understand the real content of the communication. Recognition of the communication aspects of suicidal behavior facilitates a more accurate evaluation of the various factors in the situation and allows for a more appropriate and helpful response.

The Worker in Suicide Prevention

The Effect of the Suicidal Communication

The suicidal behavior can further be understood in terms of the effect upon the recipients of the communication. For example, the communications may arouse feelings of sympathy, anxiety, anger, hostility, etc., in family or friends. Similar feelings may be aroused within the worker unless he can anticipate and counteract such reactions in himself. A universal tendency of which the worker must be aware is the desire to be omnipotent. Then (but only then) he would be able to solve all the problems and meet all of the demands of every patient. Intensely dependent patients attribute tremendous powers to the potential rescuer.

Many suicidal situations will arouse within the worker feelings of anxiety and self-doubt regarding his adequacy to handle the critical situations. While a moderate level of anxiety is appropriate, too much anxiety may seriously hamper the worker, especially if it is transmitted to the patient who, at this point, is depending upon the worker to help him solve his problems. The suicidal person who feels helpless and lost, perceiving excess anxiety in the worker, may lose his hope in the possibility of being helped. As in other aspects of life, suicide prevention workers develop confidence and poise with training and experience.

Feelings about Death

Death is a part of life and living, but in our culture it has always been surrounded by powerful taboos. These taboos and the feelings they arouse may affect the worker and even interfere in the interaction with the patient, unless the worker is sensitive to his own feelings about death. Whatever his own feelings, the worker must avoid any tendencies toward moralistic attitudes toward death and suicide. The worker's point of view within the professional situation must be that death is to be prevented, if possible; but he should recognize the existence and merits of other viewpoints.

Basic Principles of Suicide Prevention

The following comments are offered as guidelines for effective and comfortable functioning in working with suicidal persons. It it, of course, impossible to anticipate every situation.

In most cases, suicidal crises will go through several stages in resource utilization. In the early stages, the person first comes to the attention of family, relatives and friends. In the second stage, he may come into contact with front-line resources, such as family physician, clergyman, police, lawyers, school personnel, and public health nurses. If the suicidal tendencies persist, the next line of resources is called into play, the professional person and agency. The final resource may be the hospital. The professions involved will include psychiatry, psychology, psychiatric social work, and psychiatric nursing. Agencies in the community most often involved will be mental hospitals, general hospitals, psychiatric clinics, social work agencies and various service agencies such as family service, vocational rehabilitation, and employment offices. Probably, with the current development of community mental health centers and the movement toward more immediate response to both physical and emotional illnesses, the professional persons and agencies will be contacted earlier and more directly.

Recently, suicide prevention services have been started in various cities throughout the country. They are characterized by two essential components, no-waiting service and twenty-four hour availability. They offer varying degrees of service, but primarily they all have in common working on the telephone. Many suicidal persons will no doubt be contacting these specialized suicide prevention centers.

The handling of a telephone call from suicidal persons generally involves five steps. They may or may not occur concomitantly.

1. Establishing a relationship, maintaining contact, and obtaining information.
2. Identification and clarification of the focal problem(s).

3. Evaluation of the suicidal potential.
4. Assessment of strength and resources.
5. Formulation of a therapy plan and mobilization of patients' and others' resources.

Each of the steps is discussed in detail below.

Establishing a Relationship, Maintaining Contact, and Obtaining Information:

In general, the worker should be patient, interested, self-assured, hopeful, and knowledgeable. He will want to communicate by his attitude that the person has done the right thing in calling and that the worker is able and willing to help. By the fact of his call, the patient has indicated a desire for help with his problems. He should be accepted without challenge or criticism and allowed to tell his story in his own way, the worker confining himself to listening carefully to the information volunteered. The response, both in terms of attitude and tone on the telephone, will make a significant impact.

Sometimes, because the patient will not have a clear idea of the agency's functions, it will be necessary to make clear the services offered. For example, the patient may request financial aid or a home visit, and if these are not part of the service, this must be clearly stated.

A call should be initiated with a clear identification of the worker, and a request for the name and telephone number of the caller. Names and phone numbers of interested other persons such as family, physicians, close friends, or others who might be possible resources in the situation should also be obtained. The worker's immediate goal is to obtain information to be used in an evaluation of the suicidal potentiality. This is usually best accomplished by asking direct, specific questions about his suicidal feelings and plans. For example, How do you plan to commit suicide? Have you pills or gun? When? etc. It is the patient's reason for calling, and to talk about it without undue anxiety is helpful in reducing the patient's own anxiety about his suicidal impulses.

Identification and Clarification of Focal Problems

The suicidal patient often displays a profound sense of confusion, chaos and disorganization. He is unclear about his main problem and has become lost in details. One of the most important services of the worker is to help the patient recognize and order the central and the secondary problems. For example, a woman caller presented a profusion of symptoms with feelings of worthlessness, despair, and inadequacy, saying she was not a good mother, she could not manage her housework, and her family would be better off without her. All this was accompanied by incessant weeping. Questioning revealed that her main problem lay in her relationships with her husband. A statement to this effect provided her with an authoritative definition of her central conflict and she was now able to address herself to this identified problem more effectively.

In some instances the caller may be clear about his central problem, but indicates that he has exhausted all his own alternatives for solution. The worker, as an objective outsider, might be able to provide a number of additional alternatives for the patient to consider.

Evaluation of Suicide Potential

The suicide potential refers to the degree of probability that the patient may kill himself in the immediate or relatively near future. A number of criteria to evaluate suicide potentiality have been developed out of research and experience at the Los Angeles Suicide Prevention Center. Suicidal potentiality will vary in terms of lethality from minimal, in which there is no danger of loss of life, to maximal, in which the possibility of death occurring is great and immediate.

As soon as the worker begins to talk with a suicidal caller, the worker has assumed some responsibility for preventing the suicide. To do so the worker must have an accurate evaluation of the lethal risk within the suicidal behavior. The plan of action formulated by the worker will depend upon the evaluation of the suicidal risk, plus an appraisal of the patient's focal problem, his personality and available resources. The criteria for evaluation of suicide potential follow:

1. *Age and sex.* Both statistics and experience have indicated that the suicide rate for committed suicide rises with increasing age, and that men are more likely to kill themselves than women. A communication from an older male tends to be most dangerous; from a young female, least dangerous. Young people do kill themselves, even if the original aim may be to manipulate and control other people and not to die. Age and sex thus offer a general framework for evaluating the

suicidal situation, but each case requires further individual appraisal, in which the criteria which follow are most useful.

2. *Suicide plans.* This is probably the most significant of the criteria of suicide potentiality. Three main elements should be considered in appraising the suicide plan. These are (a) the lethality of the proposed method, (b) availability of the means, and (c) specificity of the details. A method involving a gun or jumping or hanging is of higher lethality than one which depends on the use of pills or wrist cutting. If the gun is at hand, the threat of its use must be taken more seriously than when the person talks about shooting himself but has no gun immediately available. In addition, if the person indicates by many specific details that he has spent time and made preparations, such as changing a will, writing notes, collecting pills, bought a gun, and set a time, the seriousness of the suicidal risk rises markedly.

Another factor in the rating of the suicide plan arises when the details are obviously bizarre. Further evaluation of the plan will depend in large degree upon the patient's psychiatric diagnosis. A psychotic person with the idea of suicide is a high risk and may make a bizarre attempt as a result of psychotic ideation.

3. *Stress.* Information about the precipitating stress usually is obtained in answer to the question, Why are you calling at this time? Typical precipitating stresses are losses, such as: loss of a loved person by death, divorce or separation; loss of job, money, prestige or status; loss of health through sickness, surgery or accident; threat of prosecution, criminal involvement or exposure. etc. Sometimes increased anxiety and tension appear as a result of success, such as promotion on the job and increased responsibilities. Stress must always be evaluated from the patient's point of view and not from the worker's or society's point of view. What might be considered minimal stress by a worker might be felt as severe for the patient. The relationship noted between stress and symptoms (next criterion) is useful in evaluating prognosis. In general, if stress and symptoms are great, the action response of the worker must be high. In contrast, if symptoms are severe, but stress is low, either the story may be incomplete or the person is chronically unstable and will give a history of prior similar crises in his life.

4. *Symptoms.* Suicidal symptoms occur in many different psychological states. Among the most common are depression, psychosis, and agitation. Evidence of a severe depressive state may be elicited with

questions about sleep disorder, loss of appetite, weight loss, social withdrawal, loss of interest, apathy and despondency, severe feelings of hopelessness and helplessness, and feelings of physical and psychological exhaustion. Psychotic states will be characterized by delusions, hallucinations, loss of contact or disorientation, or highly unusual ideas and experiences. Agitated states will show tension, anxiety, guilt, shame, poor impulse control and feelings of rage, anger, hostility and revenge. Of most significance is the state of agitated depression in which the person may feel that he is unable to tolerate the pressure of his feelings and anxieties and exhibits marked tension, fearfulness, restlessness, and pressure of speech. The patient feels he must act in some direction in order to obtain some relief from his feelings. Alcoholics, homosexuals, and drug addicts tend to be high suicidal risks.

5. *Resources.* The patient's environmental resources are often critical in determining whether or not the patient will live. Inquiry should be for resources which can be used to support him through the severe suicidal crisis. These may consist of family, relatives, close friends, physician or clergymen. If the patient is already in contact with a therapeutic agency or a professional therapist, the first consideration should be the possibility of referral back to the therapist or agency. Another resource may be the patient's work, especially when it provides him with self-esteem and gratifying relationships. Related to this is the patient's financial status which may influence the availability and location of immediate physical and psychological care.

Sometimes the patient and family try to keep the suicidal situation a secret, or even to deny its existence. As a general rule this attempt at secrecy and denial must be vigorously counteracted and the suicidal situation dealt with openly and frankly. A general principle is that it is usually better both for the worker and for the patient when the responsibility for a suicidal patient is shared by as many people as possible. This gives the patient the feeling he lacks, that others are interested and ready to help him. Where there are no apparent sources of support, the situation should be considered more ominous. The same evaluation may be applied when resources are available but have become exhausted or hostile, as when family and friends have turned away and now refuse to be concerned with the suicidal patient. In most cases people respond to crises and will help if given an opportunity to do so.

6. *Life style.* This criterion of the person's general functioning refers

to a stable versus an unstable style of life, and includes an evaluation of the suicidal behavior of the patient as acute or chronic. The stable person will report a consistent work history, stable marital and family relationships, and no history of prior suicidal behavior. If serious attempts were made in the past, the current suicidal situation may usually be rated more dangerous. The unstable personality may include severe character disorders, borderline psychotics, and persons with repeated difficulties in main areas of life functioning, such as interpersonal relationships and employment. Acute suicidal behavior may be found in either a stable or an unstable personality; chronic suicidal behavior is found only in an unstable person. With stable persons undergoing a suicidal crisis, usually in reaction to a specific stress, the worker should be highly responsive, active and invested. With unstable persons, the worker generally should be slower and more thoughtful, reminding the caller that he has weathered similar crises in the past. The main goal will be to help him through another crisis, to restore order, and to help him stay in an interpersonal relationship with a stable person or resource.

7. *Communication aspects.* The communication aspects of the suicidal situations are revealing. The most important question is whether or not communication still exists between the suicidal person and other people. The most alarming signal is when communication with the suicidal person has been completely severed. This can be an indication to the worker that the suicidal person has lost hope in any possibility of rescuing activity.

The form of the communication may be significant. In type, the communication may be either verbal or nonverbal, and, in content, it may be either direct or indirect. A serious problem in the suicidal situation occurs when the person engages in nonverbal and indirect communication. These "action communications" imply that the interchange between the suicidal person and others around him is unclear and frequently raises the probability of acting out of the suicidal impulses. In addition, if the recipient of the communication tends to deny the existence of things which upset him, it may be very difficult for him to appreciate or even recognize the suicidal nature of the communications. In general, one of the primary goals of the worker is to open up and clarify the communications among all who are involved.

The content of the communications may be directed to one or more significant persons in his environment with accusations, expressions of hostility, blame, and implied and overt demands for changes in behavior and feelings on the part of the others. Other communications may express feelings of guilt, inadequacy, worthlessness, or indications of strong anxiety and tension. When the communication is directed to specific persons, the reactions of these persons are important in the evaluation of the suicidal danger. These reactions are detailed in the following section.

8. *Reactions of significant other.* The significant other may be judged by the worker either as non-helpful, or even injurious, in the situation and therefore no possible assistance for the patient; or he may be seen as helpful and a significant resource for rescue. The nonhelpful significant others either reject the patient or deny the suicidal behavior itself and withdraw both psychologically and physically from continued communication. The significant other may resent the increased demands, the insistence on gratification of dependency needs, the dictum to change his behavior. In other cases, one may see helpless, indecisive and ambivalent behavior on the part of the significant other and the strong feeling that he does not know what the next step is and has given up. This latter reaction of hopelessness gives the suicidal person the feeling that aid is not available from a previously dependable source and may increase the patient's own feelings of hopelessness.

By contrast, a helpful reaction from the significant other is one in which the significant other recognizes the communication, is aware of the problem that needs to be dealt with and seeks help for the patient. This is an indication to the patient that his communications are being attended to and that someone is doing somthing to provide help for him.

9. *Medical status.* The medical situation of the patient may reveal additional important information for evaluating the suicidal potentiality. The patient, for example, may be suffering from a chronic, debilitating illness which has involved considerable change in self-image and self-concept. For persons with chronic illness, the relationship with their physician, their family or a hospital will be of most importance. It is a positive sign if the patient continues to see these as resources for help.

The patient may be suffering from ungrounded fears of a fatal illness, such as cancer or brain tumor, and indicate a preoccupation with death and dying. There may be a history of many repeated unsuccessful experiences with doctors or a pattern of failure in previous therapy. These symptoms are of importance because of their possible effect on the significant others and doctors, exhausting them as resources for the patient.

In general, no single criterion need be alarming, with the possible exception of the one: having a very lethal and specific plan for suicide. Rather, the evaluation of suicidal potential should be based on the general pattern of all the above criteria within the individual case. For example, feelings of exhaustion and loss of resources might well have different implications in two patients of different ages. Thus, a 25-year-old married man stated that he was tired, depressed, and was having vague ideas about committing suicide by driving into a freeway abutment. There was no history of prior suicidal behavior. He reported difficulty in his marriage and talked of separation, but he was still in contact with his wife and was still able to work on a job that he had for many years. This case was considered a low suicide risk. A contrasting case of high risk was a 64-year-old man with a history of alcoholism who reported he had made a serious suicide attempt one year ago and was saved when someone unexpectedly walked in and found him comatost. He recounted a history of three failures in marriage, and many job changes in the past year. He further stated that his physical health had been failing, that he had no family left and he was thinking of killing himself with a gun he had in his house.

Assessment of Patient's Strengths and Resources

It is as important to assess the patient's strengths and resources as it is to evaluate the pathological aspects of the picture. Frequently the patient will present alarming serious negative feelings and behaviors. These may be mitigated, however, by a number of positive features still present within the situation. For example, one indication of important internal resources may be the patient's reaction to the worker's first attempts to focus the interview. If the patient is able to respond to the worker, accepting suggestions and directions, this is an important hopeful sign. Improvement in mood and thinking within the course of one interview is a positive sign and indicates the patient's ability to respond to proffered help.

Formulation of a Therapeutic Plan and Mobilization of Patients' and Others' Resources

The plan formulated for the patient will be determined by the evaluation of the patient's suicidal status and the information obtained about him and his resources. In general, those cases with the higher suicidal potential will require the most activity on the part of the worker. An evaluation of high suicide potential in a situation which appears out of control will usually require immediate hospitalization. In our experience, however, only ten percent of the cases require this action. Family or close friends should be contacted to help bring the situation under control and to take the patient to the hospital. They should be instructed not to leave the patient alone. Most calls received by the worker are of low suicidal risk. Some of them can be handled satisfactorily by simply providing sympathetic and understanding listening with only telephone counseling and advice.

Most cases, however, will require more action on the part of the worker, usually in the process of referring the patient to another resource in the community. The type of referral depend upon the evaluation of the problem. The referral may be to either a nonprofessional or a professional resource or to both. Although most calls are not serious in terms of suicide, the callers do have serious life problems for which they need help. The suicide call is a cry for help with these problems.

If the call comes at night, the worker should keep in mind that most problems are magnified during the nighttime hours. An immediate goal would be to help the patient get through the night. The worker should strive to get sufficient information to determine if it is a high risk emergency requiring an immediate action.

In the highly unusual event that a person is calling in the midst of his suicide attempt (1 to 2 percent of the calls), as much information as is necessary to identify the patient or the caller should be obtained and the informant should be instructed either to take the patient to an emergency hospital, to call his personal physician, to call an ambulance, or to call the police. The aim at that time is to provide the patient with immediate medical attention.

At this point it is important to note an important aspect of the worker's responsibility. The worker might make a referral for the patient to one of the resources within the community, but the moral responsibility for the patient remains his until this responsibility is assumed by the other resource. The patient is thus *transferred* rather than *referred*. The worker must not assume his responsibility has been discharged until he is assured that responsibilty for care of the patient has been accepted elsewhere.

In general, if there is any question or doubt about the evaluation of the suicidal situation of the patient, he should be referred to a professional person for a complete evaluation. A patient with a suicidal problem that is not immediately serious but who presents emotional disturbances, may be referred to a psychiatric clinic, private therapist or a family agency. Usually such resources will require a waiting period and the referral to such agencies will depend upon whether or not the patient can sustain the interim period. A resource book showing available psychiatric and social agencies in the community is especially useful.

In suicide prevention, there will always appear, despite experience and knowledge, some cases which will arouse anxiety and tension in the worker. The most constructive way to handle these feelings is through informal discussions and consultation with colleagues which generally provide at least two measures of help. Not only is there a sharing of anxiety and responsibility, but there is benefit from discussion of the problem. Regular meetings for training films, lectures by professionals who have had special experience, or case presentations, help maintain morale and improve service. Comments on the problem cases of other workers should be directed toward evaluating the difficulties and offering constructive help. Every worker should be prepared for some failures. A recommended method for handling the grief experienced by workers when the suicide of a caller could not be prevented is to have a conference about the case in the spirit of mutual sympathy and support, and with the hope of learning more. In its many aspects suicide is still an enigma and there is much to be learned.

Resources

The following are detailed suggestions about general and community resources for use in suicidal situations. Any one or combinations of these resources should be considered as imaginatively and constructively as possible. The worker should not allow himself to be constrained by conventional practices. In general, the resources will be of two types, nonprofessional and professional.

1. *Nonprofessional Resources*

a. *Family.* The family is often neglected as a resource but is one of the most valuable at the time of crisis. The patient should be encouraged to discuss his situation and problems with his family. If it is considered important that someone be with the patient during the crisis, the family members should be called and apprised of the situation even though the patient may be reluctant. The patient is usually informed first that his family will be called. Also, the family must be involved in accepting responsibilities for the emergency and in helping the patient get the treatment which has been recommended.

b. *Friends.* Close friends often can be used in the same way families have been used. For example, the patient can be encouraged to have a friend stay with him during a difficult period. The friend may also be helpful in talking things out and in giving a feeling of support.

c. *Family physician.* People often turn to their family doctors for help and physicians often serve as supportive authority figures. The patient usually has a good relationship with his doctor and should be encouraged to discuss his problems with him. Physicians can also be helpful in cases where medication or hospitalization is required.

d. *Clergy.* If the caller is close to his church he should be encouraged to discuss his situation with his clergyman.

e. *Employer.* When the patient's occupation is involved and there is considerable question about his feelings of self-esteem because of vocational difficulties, the patient can be encouraged to talk about these difficulties with his employer.

f. *Police.* In metropolitan areas police should be utilized only in cases of clear and immediate emergency, e.g. if the suicide attempt is about to occur or has occurred. The patient may need prompt medical attention and the police are often the ones who can procure it for him most quickly. The police are able to take the responsibility for involvement with a patient and may hospitalize when necessary. It should be remembered, however, that the police are not to be used simply as an ambulance or transportation system. As a general rule, the police should be involved as little as possible, but when the decision to use them is made it should be carried through with firmness and dispatch. The two main criteria will be when the patient is helpless and hurt. In small cities the police may be involved as a prime resource for anyone in trouble.

g. *Emergency hospital.* Usually the patient or his family or the caller will know of private emergency hospitals in his area. The worker should know about city and county hospitals available for emergency medical treatment hospitalization. The police will generally use city and county hospitals.

2. *Professional Resources.*

a. *Own agency.* The worker may wish to refer the patient to his own agency in those cases where it is felt there is a high suicide potential and where there is need for more intensive, careful further evaluation. Giving the patient an appointment gives the patient a task and a purpose to his immediate future. This resource, of course, can be used only when the agency includes facilities for personal interview and evaluation.

b. *Social work agencies and community psychiatric clinics.* In those cases where the suicide danger has been evaluated as low or perhaps not even the primary problem, a referral to a family service agency or community psychiatric clinic can be considered. These are often the treatment medium of choice for patients in whom the underlying problem may be seen as marital discord, family conflict, or chronic personal and social maladjustment. The worker should be familiar with the social work agencies or community psychiatric clinics within the community and referrals can be made to those near the patient. Often, a referral to an agency which works primarily with persons of the patient's own religion is more desirable. Other considerations are fees and hours which will be compatible for the patient.

c. *Private therapists.* Some calls are from people looking for psychiatric treatment. The worker should be familiar with private therapists for appropriate recommendation in such cases. If the patient indicates that he is already in treatment, he should be encouraged to return to his own therapist.

d. *Psychiatric hospital.* If the community contains a psychiatric hospital or a general hospital with a psychiatric ward where patients can be hospitalized, a liaison with such facilities is most important.

Generally, referral to such a resource is made when it is thought the patient is so disturbed that he might seriously harm himself or others, and/or he is so disorganized he can no longer exercise judgment or direction of his affairs. It might be necessary to have family or friends take the patient to the hospital if the patient himself is incapable of getting there.

Some Typical Calls

Following are some illustrations of what may be considered typical calls. A description is given of the caller and the problem presented and suggestions will be made for the handling of the call. It should be remembered that these are examples which have been generalized for teaching purposes and that calls do not always fall exactly within these given descriptions.

1. A woman, between 30 and 40 years old, calls at night saying that she does not understand why she feels so depressed. She states she is alone, complains of not being able to sleep, having troubled thoughts and feels that she needs to talk to someone. Sometimes she will say that she really does not want to kill herself but she has had suicidal thoughts over many months or years. She may be agitated, depressed, weeping, as if she is having a hysterical breakdown. She may be demanding and asks what can be done to help her right now because she feels she is not able to get through the night. Questioning will reveal she has had many similar episodes before. Probably she is reacting to some interpersonal conflict such as an argument with a family member or close friend.

It is best to listen patiently and wait for the opportunity to point out realistically that things look worse at night, but that is not the best time when she can get help for herself. She should be advised to call her doctor or social work agency or clinic in the morning so as to arrange a program of help for herself. It may be helpful to suggest that she call a close friend or relative to come and be with her during this difficult night.

2. A woman sounds as if she were between 20 and 35 years old, but who will not identify herself. She asks what can the Suicide Prevention Center do for a person who does not want to live anymore, and generally takes a challenging position. The caller sounds controlled, makes vague allusions to a long-standing problem, and wants

to know what you can do about it. Frequently these no-name callers are either in psychotherapy or have been recently interrupted.

The worker should point out that the caller has responsibility to clarify his request and cooperate if he is to receive help. You must know who he is and about his situation before you can assist him. If he tells you he has a therapist, and who he is, you should refer him back to the therapist. Tell him that you will call the therapist to notify him that the patient had called you.

3. A woman between 40 and 55 calls about herself, complaining that she is very depressed, feels lonely and tired, and feels that no one is interested in her. She talks about many physical and medical problems. She says that she feels her doctor is not helping her enough and that her husband is not paying enough attention to her. She will say that she feels like her life is over, and there is no point in continuing to live.

An effort should be made to talk with the husband and to discuss with him how his wife is feeling. Both the patient and the husband should be encouraged to talk with the family physician at the first opportunity about the patient's depression. You may offer to call the physician, too, in order to enlist his aid. If none of these resources seems available, the patient may be asked to come in for an appointment.

4. A man between 18 and 30 sounds evasive and anxious on the phone and is reluctant to give his name. He talks about having a problem which he is hesitant to identify, and states he is calling for help because the only solution he can think of is to kill himself. His suicide plan will be an impulsive one, like smashing his car up on the freeway, or cutting himself with a razor blade. This man often has a personal problem about which he feels guilty, such as homosexuality.

This patient should be encouraged to seek help for himself. You should commend him for having done the right thing in calling you as a beginning effort to get help for himself. You might suggest a resource where he might go, such as a psychiatric clinic, private therapist, physician, or school counselor.

5. A man between 25 and 40 complains that his life is just a mess because of his bungling. He talks about having gotten himself into such a jam, either financially or with his family or on the job,

that he feels the only way out is to kill himself. Often he will be reacting to a specific, recent setback in his life.

He should be told that he is reacting to a specific stress, and that he needs help with that particular problem about which he feels helpless and hopeless. He should be reminded that he was able to function well before he had this setback, that he is suffering from a depression which is most often time-limited and temporary and that he needs help to get back on his feet again. He should be encouraged to come in for an appointment, and every effort made to help him resolve the stress and get through the crisis.

6. A man about 50 or so sounds very depressed and discouraged and seems apologetic about calling and troubling you. He may complain about a physical problem which has prevented his working, and feels now that he is beyond help. His general feelings about himself are that he is old and infirm and a burden on others. When asked what his suicidal thoughts are he talks about specific plans for killing himself.

Friends, family and resources should be mobilized and involved. The patient should be told that help is available to him. He should be told to come in for an appointment and his family should be impressed with the need to follow through. If he fails to come in, then he should be called back and contact maintained until someone takes responsibility for treatment of such a high suicidal risk.

7. A family member or friend calls about a person who is described as depressed, withdrawn, or has shown some behavioral or personality change. The patient may have told them that he is planning to kill himself and even discussed a specific plan with them, or he may have generally talked about wanting to end his life. The caller is asking how serious the situation is and what he should do.

The caller should be advised to contact the patient and let him know he is concerned about him and trying to get help. He should be told to have the patient call you, so that the patient will have the feeling that help is being obtained for him, and also, you will have an opportunity to evaluate the situation with the patient. You should maintain your contact with the initial caller and keep him apprised of what is happening, maintaining him as a resource to help, if need be. The recommendation to the patient will depend on the evaluation of the lethal potentiality.

8. The caller is a neighbor or friend and is concerned about some-one he knows. He may be reluctant to identify himself or to involve himself in any responsibility but requests that you do something about the person he is concerned about. He is not able to give too much detail or information about the situation which concerns him.

You should get as much information as you can and encourage him to let the person know that he is concerned for him and to advise the patient to call you. You should point out that it would be unrealistic for you simply to call someone without being able to say who notified you. The caller should be told that it is his responsibility to be in-volved if he is really concerned about a person who is suicidal.

9. A physician, minister, police officer, or similar person in a posi-tion of responsibility calls about a case. Frequently, the call is about someone who has just been rescued after a suicide attempt.

Get as much information as possible to evaluate the situation. If the patient is still threatening suicide, hospitalization should be con-sidered. If the patient seems calmed down and under control, then he should be encouraged to seek professional help. Your informant should be encouraged to demonstrate his continued interest in the patient and offer counseling.

10. The caller tells you about a neighbor or family member who is being physically restrained from attempting suicide and the patient cannot be left unattended. The patient is described as psychotic and determined to kill himself.

The caller should be advised to take the patient to the nearest psychiatric hospital or to the psychiatric unit of the county general hospital. It should be emphasized that harmful drugs or objects should be removed from the patient's environment and someone should al-ways be with him.

11. In the unusual event that you get a call from someone who is attempting suicide while telling you about it, you should keep the person on the phone. Get his name, phone number, address, and information about his attempt. Try to learn specifically what he has ingested or what he is doing. Call the police and identify yourself, give them all the pertinent information and ask them to investigate.

Appendix A
EXAMPLES OF WORKSHEETS

MODEL PHONE WORKSHEET
(John Hinkle, Ph.D.)

CALLER'S NAME_____Time ____(AM)__(PM)_____

1. Statement of problem:

Date _____
Day _____
Volunteer _____
Length of call _____
Sex of caller: M_____ F_____

2. Caller's level of stress, anxiety, suicide potential (include symptoms of and degree of seriousness):

3. Primary Diagnosis (place a "1" in appropriate grid)

   Secondary Diagnosis (place a "2" in appropriate grid)

Answer following items if given by caller:

Phone _____
Age _____
Residence _____
Location call was made from _____
_____
Student _____ Nonstudent _____
Year _____

	(1) Lack of information about self	(2) Lack of information about environment	(3) Conflict with self	(4) Conflict with significant other	(5) Lack of skill
Social (1) Emotional (2) Educational (3)					

MARITAL STATUS (check one)

____Single ____Married ____Divorced
____Widowed ____Separated

4. Contacts volunteer made concerning call as well as referrals, suggestions, recommendations, etc.

5. Follow-up information

   Agency _____
   Personnel _____
   Phone No. _____

6. COMMENTS:

_____Referred to other agency for treatment
_____Treatment in progress (continuing client)
_____Treatment terminated by client prior to completion
_____Treatment completed during phone interview
_____Treatment completed; additional type of service recommended.

PHONE ANSWERING FORM

Student Services   NO. _____
University of Illinois SEE ALSO NO. _____

Date _____   NAME OF CLIENT _____
Time _____AM/PM   Address _____
                            Age _____ Phone _____ Other info. _____
                            Caller's name _____
                                        (if different from above)
                            Address _____ Phone _____
                            Relationship to client _____

TYPE OF CALL

_____Medical   _____Drug info   _____Employment
_____Legal   _____Bad trip   _____Housing
_____Psychiatric   _____Suicide   _____General info
_____Counsel   _____Transportation   _____Follow-up call
     (general)   _____Runaway (under 18)   _____Other_____
                      _____Missing person (over 18)

Describe problem _____
_____
_____
_____

Action taken:
_____ Had general conversation _____
_____ Gave advice _____
_____

_____ Referral to:
            Name   *Address/Agency*   *Phone*
        _____   _____   _____
        _____   _____   _____
        _____   _____   _____

_____ Other _____

FOLLOW-UP CALLS

Call In	Out	Date	Name	Phone	Regarding	Initial
___	___	_____	_____	_____	_____	___
___	___	_____	_____	_____	_____	___
___	___	_____	_____	_____	_____	___

Evaluation (by supervisor and/or director) _____
_____
_____
_____

                                                    Initial

HELP LINE
University of Utah

_____

Month   Day   Year

Male   Female

Time call started _____

Time call ended _____

Student at: U of U   High School

Other: _____

Referred to: _____

Weather:

    Clear Cloudy Rain Snow

Phone   In Person

Age ____ Reported Guessed ____

Jr. High   Not attending School

Year in School: _____

SCHOOL

_____Grades

_____Rules, registration, etc.

_____Other

INTERPERSONAL RELATIONSHIPS

_____Parents

_____Roommates

_____Boyfriend—girlfriend

_____Loneliness, poor social life

_____Other

PSYCHOLOGICAL—MEDICAL

_____General emotional problems

_____Suicide threat

_____Drugs, crisis

_____Drugs, information

_____Birth control information

_____Pregnancy

_____Other

LEGAL—FINANCIAL

_____Money shortage

_____Job security

_____Legal aid

_____Housing

_____Draft

_____Other

MISCELLANEOUS

_____Prank

_____Wrong number

_____Information about HELP

_____Hung up without a response

_____Other

    1   2   3   4   5   6   7   8   9

_____

Not urgent   Extremely urgent

PHONE ANSWERING FORM
RoadHouse
Colorado State University

Time _____(AM) (PM)

Date _____

Day _____

Volunteer _____

Length of call _____

1. Statement of problem:

2. Caller's level of stress, anxiety, suicide potential
   (include symptoms of and degree of seriousness).

3. Contacts volunteer made concerning call as well as referrals, suggestions, recommendations, etc.

4. Sex: M_____   F_____

5. Answer following items if given by caller during call:
   Phone _____ Residence _____
   Age _____ Location call was made from _____
   _____
   Class _____ Student _____ Nonstudent _____

6. Follow-up information:
   Agency _____
   Personnel _____
   Phone No. _____

7. COMMENTS:

Y.E.S. PHONE FORM

Youth Emergency Service   Form No. _____
Minneapolis—St. Paul   See also No. _____

Date _____

DAY OF WEEK
__Sunday
__Monday
__Tuesday
__Wednesday
__Thursday
__Friday
__Saturday

CALL WAS PRIMARILY
__Information
__Referral
__Counseling

CATEGORY
__Alternatives
__Depression
__Drug—currently high
__Drug—related problem
__Drug—information
__Employment
__Entertainment
__Family
__Food/Clothing
__Housing
__Legal—Civil
__Legal—Criminal
__Loneliness
__Medical—abortion
__Medical—emergency
__Medical—free/ lowcost
__Medical—birth control

__Suicide
__Transportation
__Veterinary
__Welfare
__Other_____

WAS CALL REFERRED?
__Yes
__No

TIME OF CALL
__1AM-6AM
__6AM-10AM
__10AM-2PM
__2PM-6PM
__6PM-10PM
__10PM-1AM

AGE OF CALLER
__17 and under
__18-24
__25 and over
__Unknown

SEX OF CALLER
__Female
__Male

LOCATION OF CALL
Mpls.
__City, So.
__City, No.
Mpls. suburbs
__West
__South
__North

Check if possible repeat-caller _____

CALLER INFORMATION
(Complete only when necessary)

First Name _____

Address _____

Phone _____
(get address and phone only in emerg.)

Caller's Situation:

_____
_____
_____
_____
_____
_____
_____

Volunteer's Response:

_____
_____
_____
_____
_____
_____

___Medical—dental
___Medical—pregnancy
___Medical—V.D.
___Medical—other
___Military—draft
___Military—in service
___Military—other
___Political
___Relationship—
straight
___Relationship—gay
___Runaway
___Sexuality

St. Paul
___City
___Suburbs
Other
___Out state
___Other
___Unknown
LENGTH OF
CALL
___Up to 5 min.
___5 to 20 min.
___20 to 40 min.
___over 40 min.

Referral: (Most important
for C.I.T., ambulance,
other emergencies)

Name _____

Clinic/agency _____

Phone _____

Y.E.S. Volunteer's Name _____

OPEN LINE CALLER INFORMATION

Open Line, Inc.   A.M.

Ames, Iowa   Time _____ P.M.

Listener's Full Name _____ Date _____ ____ ___

                                          month   day   yr

Day
1 Sunday
2 Monday
3 Tuesday
4 Wednesday
5 Thursday
6 Friday
7 Saturday

Problem(s)
01 "Put-on"
02 Request for specific volunteer
03 Boy-girl relations: wants date
04 Boy-girl relations: dating friction
05 Dating: other
06 Loneliness
07 Family problems: parent-child
08 Family problems: spouses
09 Family problems: siblings
10 Family problems: other
11 Race relations
12 Other interpersonal problems
13 Suicide
14 Alcohol
15 Drugs: experience
16 Drugs: information
17 Drugs: legal
18 Drugs: illegal
19 Birth control

Type of Contact
1 Phone-in
2 Walk-in
3 Phone-out
4 Appointment

Sex of Caller
1 Male
2 Female

Persons calling
1 One caller
2 More than one

Focus of Concern
1 Caller personally
2 Caller's associate

Length of Contact
(in minutes)

_____

Prior Contact
0 Unknown
1 No
2 Yes—with whom? _____

_____

Age Group
1 Estimated
2 Certain

1 Grade school
2 Jr. high school
3 High school
4 College
5 Mature student
6 Young adult
7 Middle age
8 Late middle age
9 Senior citizen

Initial Distress of Caller
1 Not at all distressed
2 Possibly slightly distressed
3 Moderate distress
4 Highly distressed
5 Exceptionally high distress

Anonimity
1 No name
2 First name requested—not given
3 First name requested—given
4 First name volunteered
5 First name of self and others given
6 More complete information

131

20 Pregnancy
21 Abortion
22 Sex information
23 Other medical
24 Studying
25 University information
26 Open Line information
27 Community information
28 Mental health information
29 Employment
30 Financial
31 Legal
32 Draft
33 Runaway
34 General dissatisfaction
35 Other _____

Future Contact
1 Certain
2 Probable
3 Referred to mental health agency
4 Referred to other agency for information
5 Referred for special activities
6 Terminated—no future contact expected

Appendix B
SAMPLES OF PROBLEMS HANDLED

HOTLINE CALLS FOR ONE YEAR*
TYPES OF CALLS

	Male	Female	Total	%
Drug Dependency	58	59	117	(11.5)**
Alcohol	21	14	35	3.4
Intoxicated at time of call	17	10	27	
Other drugs (Speed, LSD, etc.)	37	45	82	8.1
Intoxicated at time of call	20	16	36	
Interpersonal Problems	96	225	321	(31.6)
Dating	24	64	88	8.7
Marital discord	3	64	67	6.6
Family problems	14	25	39	3.8
Lonely and depressed	33	54	87	8.6
Suicidal	12	12	24	2.4
Feeling inadequate	10	6	16	1.6
Sexual Problems	16	20	36	3.5
Pregnancy	11	18	29	2.9
Homosexuality	5	2	7	.7
Informational	116	149	265	(26.1)
Inquiry about phone service	44	49	93	9.1
Campus Information	60	93	153	15.0
Draft information	4	3	7	.7
Legal information	8	4	12	1.2
Miscellaneous	109	129	278	(27.3)
Academic problems	11	19	30	2.9
Health problems	8	27	35	3.4
Religious concerns	4	2	6	.6
Wanted to talk to someone	57	66	123	12.1
Crank calls	29	15	44	4.3
Hung up before talking	?	?	40	3.9

GRAND TOTALS

	Winter Qtr.	Spring Qtr.	Summer Qtr.	Fall Qtr.	Total	%
Male	169	61	13	175	418	41.3
Female	163	128	39	207	542	53.6
Unidentified	23	4	2	23	52	5.1

TIME OF CALLS

Time	%	Time	%
6-7 PM	10.0	12-1 AM	11.9
7-8 PM	12.1	1-2 AM	6.1
8-9 PM	13.6	2-3 AM	4.1
9-10 PM	11.1	3-4 AM	2.4
10-11 PM	15.2	4-5 AM	1.7
11-12 PM	10.9	5-6 AM	.9

LENGTH OF CALLS

Length	%	Length	%
30 minutes or less	73.0	2 hours to 4 hours	4.3
30 minutes to 1 hour	12.6	4 hours or longer	.4
1 hour to 2 hours	9.7		

DAY OF THE WEEK

Day	%	Day	%
Sunday	10.6	Thursday	11.7
Monday	13.7	Friday	17.3
Tuesday	15.5	Saturday	16.2
Wednesday	15.0		

MONTH

Month	%	Month	%
January	10.8	July	3.5
February	16.9	August	.8
March	8.0	September	1.2
April	10.3	October	17.3
May	8.5	November	16.6
June	1.3	December	4.8

*The Hotline is listed with the University of Northern Colorado, Greeley, Colorado, 80631. The tabled figures were compiled for 1970.

**Bracketed numbers are group percentages.

STATISTICAL ANALYSIS, JULY-SEPTEMBER, 1971
Hotline
Hempstead, Manhasset, N. Y.

Category	July	August	September
Days in Operation	30	31	12
Average Calls per Night			
Fri. nights only	18.8	11.7	18.5
Sat. nights only	18.2	16.0	21.0
Total Calls	15.6	12.0	18.0
Substantive Calls	10.9	8.2	15.2
Total Calls in Month	468	372	216
Substantive Calls	326	255	183
% Substantive Calls	70%	69%	85%
Calls from Boys	120	97	57
Percent	36%	36%	30
Girls	213	169	131
Percent	64%	64%	70%
Average Caller Age (Years)	16.8	16.7	15.0
Average Call Length (Minutes)	17.5	18.0	12.7
Total Hours on Phone	94.7	78.6	37.9
Unsubstantive Calls			
Gag calls	8	7	2
Wrong numbers	4	2	1
Hang-ups	127	101	29
Type of Calls			
Family calls	15	9	18
Social problems	63	41	32
Drug problems	36	25	18
Drug emergencies	9	13	5
Suicidal involvement	5	3	1
Psychological/personal	41	33	18
Companionship/lonely	23	13	7
Pregnancy inquiries	17	23	9
V.D. information	4	5	1
Medical referrals	6	4	2
Legal problems	10	4	4
Theft/crime/steal	2	1	0
Travel/housing	6	2	1
Network inquiries	8	13	7
Drinking/alcohol	4	1	5
Smoking/tobacco	1	1	0

Category	July	August	September
Days in Operation	30	31	12
Illness/disease	0	0	0
Sexual problems	21	13	15
Crisis alert	0	1	0
Information (General)	3	4	5
Inquiries (General)	36	33	30
Runaway information	5	3	1
Festival/activities	2	4	1
Employment inquiries	1	0	0
School problems	0	1	1
Political/draft	2	4	0
Gratitude	3	2	2
Pollution	1		
Spiders	1		
Ghosts	1		
Music	2		
Funerals		1	
Lost turtle			1
	329	257	185

CALLS TO ROADHOUSE

Colorado State University
Fort Collins, Colorado

Referrals		Spring '70	Fall '70	Winter '71	Spring '71
Academic advising		1	5	5	3
Health center		10	15	33	7
Counseling center		6	11	18	12
Student housing		2	0	0	1
ASCSU		7	0	9	1
Draft		2	3	8	4
Legal aid		5	11	22	17
Police		3	1	9	7
Misc. community		7	6	36	19
UCM		0	2	14	11
Days—Shifts					
Sunday	1st	1	26	48	40
	2nd	7	28	35	25
	3rd	0	8	4	10
Monday	1st	0	51	54	35
	2nd	15	26	32	29
	3rd	0	8	18	7
Tuesday	1st	3	22	44	38
	2nd	13	48	30	36
	3rd	0	6	13	14
Wednesday	1st	6	36	41	33
	2nd	19	28	46	24
	3rd	0	8	11	17
Thursday	1st	7	32	31	42
	2nd	14	42	25	25
	3rd	2	8	16	13
Friday	1st	8	26	36	30
	2nd	16	31	26	18
	3rd	5	20	14	9
Saturday	1st	6	27	48	34
	2nd	8	22	21	19
	3rd	3	12	25	9
Categories of calls					
Drugs					
Busts		4	1	7	2
OD		0	2	4	1
Information		3	26	24	18
Bummer		1	7	9	4
Information on RoadHouse		7	37	30	13
Sex					
Pregnancy		2	16	9	7
Abortion		4	5	34	16
VD		0	1	2	5
Homosexual		1	12	23	3
Birth control		3	14	17	6

139

Referrals	Spring '70	Fall '70	Winter '71	Spring '71
Medical	5	10	19	15
Counlseling center	0	11	3	4
Depression				
Loneliness	7	14	22	17
Suicide	1	4	1	2
Social interaction				
Male-Female relationships	9	25	29	45
Legal information	8	20	39	25
Draft information	5	13	15	13
General CSU information	15	65	68	50
CSU activities	21	41	46	36
Community activities	13	36	54	51
Major changes	0	2	1	1
Class problems	1	2	9	5
Professor problems	1	1	3	3
Transportation	5	14	9	8
General rap	5	28	58	71
Crash pad	2	10	7	14
Miscellaneous	4	95	95	84
Crank calls	3	3	2	0
Alcohol	1	4	2	2
Housing	4	12	5	7
Dorm problems	1	5	8	3
Total Calls	133	515	620	514
Sex of caller				
Male	71	299	324	243
Female	62	216	296	269
Callers				
Student	75	268	325	286
Nonstudent	10	51	49	92
Don't know	48	196	246	136

AUTHOR'S INDEX

SUBJECT INDEX